Let Me Get This Off My Chest: A Breast Cancer Survivor Over-shares

By Margaret Lesh

ISBN: 0615812511
ISBN-13: 978-0615812519

ISBN: 0615812511
ISBN-13: 978-0615812519

StoryRhyme

Editor, Ellen Brock
Cover design and interior layout, Steven Lesh
StoryRhyme.com Publishing

Dedication:

To all with breasts (two *or* one), to all with no breasts, to all the survivors, and to all in treatment. This one's for all of us.

And to Steve, who's been with me every step of the way, I don't know how I would have done it without you.

Be kind whenever possible. It is always possible.
~ *Dalai Lama*

Margaret Lesh

[Contents]

Our Floating Year

**Have patience with
all things, but first
of all, with yourself.**
~ Saint Francis de Sales

The year of 2012 was largely spent waiting. Waiting for appointments. Waiting for doctors. Waiting for surgeries. Waiting for healing. We weren't "doing" things, not having much in the way of fun—in fact, quite the opposite.

One day, while I was complaining about the sucky suckiness of my sucky situation, whining about how 2012 was the year that would not stop sucking, my patient partner-in-life Steve, with a calm look on his face, said, "It's okay. 2012 is our floating year."

I got it.

Just like that. I totally got it.

2012 was like a placeholder in the scheme of our lives together. This was a temporal matter. Life would go on. Eventually.

In March of 2012, I was diagnosed with a recurrence of ductal carcinoma in situ after a routine mammogram showed cellular abnormalities.

The innocent-sounding voice on the answering machine stopped me in my tracks: "This message is for Margaret Lesh from the Radiology Department at Kaiser. We need you to come in and have some additional films taken."

I'd had countless mammograms in the past twelve years since my first occurrence; they'd all come back normal. I'm not exactly a pessimist; I prefer to think of myself as a glass-half-full kind of person, but I knew. Somehow, I knew my cancer had returned.

Steve tried to reassure me.

"Oh, it'll be fine. Don't worry."

But I did worry.

So two days after my annual screening—within perhaps two hours of the phone call from the radiology department—I was back at Kaiser with my breast up on the slab having additional films taken.

Strangely enough—and possibly because I simply hadn't had enough time to process things—I wasn't freaking out. Okay, not *too* much. My gut was a little clenched, breathing was becoming shallow. My inner mantra of "*stay calm, stay calm*" was fighting the involuntary nervous state I was in.

In short, I was calm on the outside, a mess on the inside.

Poor Lefty. For the second time in three days, my left breast (aka Lefty, the Troublemaker) was once again placed on the shelf at the Women's Center and flattened.

A few moments later, as the technician put the films up on the light box, I asked her what she'd found, making my way over to where she stood, clutching my hospital gown.

"Are there any microcalcifications?"

"Yes, there are. Right here." She pointed to a little dot of white about the size of a pencil tip. There were several dots of white in two areas of my breast.

Crap.

That was it; my suspicions were confirmed.

I dressed, collected Steve from the waiting area, and we walked down the long hall to the radiology department and its crowded waiting room, mammography films in my hand.

"I hope this doesn't take too long," I said, as we stood in line at the reception desk. The last thing I wanted was a long wait to hear my fate, to add insult to injury.

We didn't wait long. Cancer is serious business. Something most people probably don't know: one of the "perks" of cancer is always being on the stat list. Every time I have blood drawn before my appointments with my oncologist, I get to go in the stat line, bypassing all the mere mortals with their non-cancer blood tests.

Silver linings; right?

We waited a few minutes, and the nurse escorted us back to Dr. Feinstein, a pleasant-looking woman in her late thirties with wire-rimmed glasses and shoulder-length brown hair. She was sitting at her desk, and right away I noticed the open, compassionate expression on her face. My films were already up on the light box situated on the wall behind her.

"Hi, I'm Dr. Feinstein. I understand you have a history of breast cancer?"

"Yes, I was diagnosed in December of 1999."

"You had a lumpectomy?"

"Yes, and radiation."

We chatted like that for a minute or two, catching her up on my history. To let her know I was up on things and that I wouldn't have a meltdown in front of her, I said, "I saw the microcalcifications. I had them the first time."

She nodded; I saw concern in her eyes. I knew, and she knew, and I knew she knew: "it" had returned.

Her steady, reassuring gaze told me: *I'm going to take care of this for you*, and she offered, "If you want, I can do a biopsy right now."

I took a breath and looked over at Steve. He nodded.

So, just like that, in the space of a little over an hour since my arrival at Kaiser, I was preparing myself to have a breast biopsy.

Life was starting to feel a bit more real than it had three hours before.

My Biopsy 2012

There is no hope unmingled with fear, and no fear unmingled with hope.

~ *Baruch Spinoza*

"We're going to do a stereotactic biopsy procedure today," Dr. Feinstein explained.

The procedure room was very high tech. I lay down on an exam table which had a cutout for my breast, which was compressed, with the images showing up on a display monitor, enabling Dr. Feinstein and her technician assistant to zero in on the location of the microcalcifications. After first numbing my breast, she then inserted the needle and collected the tissue sample from the area. I didn't feel much, other than tugging, as the doctor withdrew the samples. When the procedure was over, Dr. Feinstein and her technician pressed towels against my breast to stop the bleeding—a side effect of the procedure—but it didn't hurt.

"You should hear by Monday," Dr. Feinstein said. "I don't think there's any way the pathology will be done tomorrow."

It was Thursday; I wanted the results immediately, but, of course, things don't work that way. This was important stuff. Medical stuff. These things take time.

We shook hands, and I felt glad to have had her as my radiologist for the day. She was much more pleasant than the doctor I'd met two years prior when I'd had a biopsy of Righty, my non-cancer breast. He wasn't as optimistic and seemed convinced I would be dropping dead soon. (I didn't.)

Leaving the radiology department, I had two choices: I could (A) worry nonstop for at least three days, waiting to hear the results; or (B) I could realize that I had no control over the situation, and it was out of my hands. Worrying would net me exactly nothing.

What do you think I chose?

Of course, I chose A. Not to say that I worried the *whole* time. Sometimes I chose the optimistic route, or I'd say to myself, "You have this whole weekend to think of yourself as normal; nothing is wrong with you until you hear otherwise." This thought would give me momentary comfort until the demons of doubt entered my head, telling me: "Don't be ridiculous. Of course it's back, silly! You saw the microcalcifications, didn't you? Of course it's cancer."

My inner self can be a real jerk sometimes.

But then I thought: *If I prepare myself mentally, at least that's half the battle; I won't be caught off guard. I won't be an emotional mess.*

Yeah, right.

Back To The Beginning Of My Story

- December 1999

Fear is a darkroom where negatives develop.
~ *Usman B. Asif*

When I was thirty-four years old, in November of 1999, a couple of weeks before Thanksgiving, I felt a lump in my left breast. I'd never been the type to be zealous about my monthly breast self-exams. They were something I did when I thought about it—maybe an occasional quick, cursory check in the shower every now and then. Here and there.

What is that? Do I feel something?

I played with a little place located at about the three o'clock position on the side of my breast. I probed it for two days, harassing poor Lefty, sometimes feeling the lump, sometimes not. Was it my imagination? It was this mysterious thing; sometimes there, if the conditions were right, like *Brigadoon**. Sitting up in bed one night, I mentioned it to Steve, who knitted his brows and felt.

"I don't feel anything," he said, making me feel slightly better for about two seconds. But then: "Wait. Yeah, I think I do."

Crap.

"It's probably nothing," I said, immediately backpedaling before things got too serious, as if by saying the words, I could have some sort of effect on reality. "I'm just being paranoid."

"Still, though, you should get it checked out," he said with an undercurrent of worry that he tried to disguise.

I was thirty-four years old, too young.

There was no history of breast cancer in my family, no real risk factors, other than that I'd had my son at thirty-two and hadn't breastfed very long. My relationship with birth control pills was irregular, so there wasn't the risk factor of having been on the Pill for too many years.

I hemmed and hawed, rolling it over in my head, trying to talk myself out of it, not wanting to take it seriously. But Steve urged me to have it examined, so I called Kaiser the next afternoon to quiet him. I told the scheduling person on the other end of the phone that I'd found a lump in my breast.

"We'd better get you in. Let's get it checked out."

She didn't seem worried, her tone was businesslike, which seemed reasonable enough. I mean, it's not like it was actually going to *be* anything.

It couldn't be.

I drove myself to the little Kaiser facility conveniently located around the corner from our house. It wasn't a full hospital like the one a few miles away, just a small satellite clinic. I can't remember the name of the doctor I saw that day. He seemed, truthfully, young and inexperienced, almost like he wasn't sure about the whole "breast" thing.

"So you're here about… A lump on your breast?" he said, in a lost, almost distracted way.

"Yes, I noticed it a few days ago. I just, you know, wanted to get it checked out. I've been feeling it a few days, then I had my husband feel it. I wasn't sure…"

I babbled nervously as the young doctor tentatively probed Lefty.

"Did you feel it?" I asked.

"I'm not sure."

His forehead bore little furrows of confusion. I reached out, feeling a little like an older woman teaching a younger man about the ways of the world, and took his hand, guiding it to where the lump was. I will never forget the way his brows arched in surprise over the tops of his glasses, like two upside down Vs.

This was not good; I was *not* experiencing warm, happy thoughts. More like: *Oh, crap.*

"I do feel something. I'm going to refer you for a mammogram."

It wasn't real *yet*. It was getting there though. Quickly. I thought about work.

What do I do? Do I file for disability if it turns out to be cancer?

The mammogram was a week away, leaving me plenty of time to stress, time to reflect, time to worry.

My thoughts, as I left Kaiser, focused on my little boy. I felt my world spinning out of control.

It couldn't be cancer.

[*Brigadoon is a Broadway musical which involved a mysterious fog-covered land that could be seen with a little magic. Steve was in his high school's production.]

My First Mammogram (Or: Now, The Hurty Part)

We experience moments absolutely free from worry. These brief respites are called panic.

~ *Cullen Hightower*

The technician at the Women's Health Center arranged my breast on the little shelf, then proceeded to compress Lefty between the blocks, instructing me to take a deep

Let Me Get This Off My Chest

breath and hold it. She took extra films of the area on the side of my breast where I'd felt the lump.

It was the opposite of fun.

"Wait here. Let me check the films."

I waited in the mammography exam room while she looked at them. She frowned.

"Did you wear deodorant today?"

Crap. I'd forgotten. One mustn't wear deodorant when having a mammogram; it does something to the machines and makes the films come out wonky. I gave her a weak smile.

"Here. Use these. Clean your underarms. We need to get all the deodorant off because it could be affecting the films."

I wiped my underarms thoroughly with the little alcohol wipes; she squeezed my breast again, taking two more pictures.

I waited as she put the films up on the light box; again she frowned.

Not good.

"Do you see something?" I asked.

She motioned me over. I clutched my robe closed and peered at the films up on display.

"Do you see those little dots there? They're micro-calcifications."

"What is that, like a calcium deposit?"

The technician nodded. "A lot of times they don't mean anything."

"But?"

"But they can be a sign of necrotic tissue. The calcifications fill in the dead areas."

"Necrotic" meant dead. I had enough medical terminology in my court reporting background to know that.

"But I'm really not supposed to say anything," she said. "You need to talk to the radiologist about this."

I could tell. She knew. She'd seen enough breasts and developed enough films. She knew.

I sat in the waiting area while she packaged up the films and then walked them to the radiology department in the next building over. It felt as if I were walking to the gas chamber or gallows. I experienced numbness as I processed the information and prepared for the worst, while hoping for the best—all of those cliché things that go through your head when you're faced with a possibly life-altering circumstance. I carried the envelopes containing the films down that long hall not knowing that my life would soon change forever.

My Son Is Two, I Can't Have Cancer

When you are a mother, you are never really alone in your thoughts. A mother always has to think twice, once for herself and once for her child.

~ *Sophia Loren*

When I'd taken that long walk to the radiology department the previous Thursday, I was sent home after waiting maybe five minutes or so. The radiologist didn't need to talk to me. At that moment, I felt elation. It was okay. I didn't have cancer!

But maybe he just didn't want to give me the bad news. Maybe he wanted to pass the buck. I'll never know why I was given false hope, but I was. I'd had a peaceful weekend, thinking all was well, and then got the call on Tuesday instructing me to come in for a consultation.

The nurse's voice on the other end of the phone was calm; no hint of urgency.

"This is standard procedure. We just need you to come in so we can go over the results of your mammogram."

Huh, I thought. *That's weird. Do they do that with everybody?*

Steve was out visiting one of his customers, so I drove myself to the doctor's appointment.

"No, it's okay. It's nothing. They just want to go over the results," I said, attempting to reassure him that he didn't need to change his work plans for me.

"I know it's okay. I just want to be there."

In the back of my head, in the back of his head, we knew something wasn't right. Sixth sense maybe?

Steve found me sitting in the waiting room; he'd made it there just in time for me to be called in. We met Dr. Ruiz, who we'd soon come to know as a serious person—stoic, not light, not funny. He handed me a pamphlet; it said something horrible like, "Treatment of Breast Cancer."

I was beginning to get very suspicious that something was going on. (Yes, I'm *that* smart.)

Dr. Ruiz gave me a quizzical look, probably sensing my confusion, and said, "Didn't anybody talk to you?"

"No. The nurse on the phone said this was standard procedure—to come in to go over mammogram results."

When I said it out loud, I realized how dumb it sounded. I think it was something called "denial." But in my defense, the whole process had been very confusing, as if one hand didn't know what the other hand was doing.

"From the films, it looks like you have ductal carcinoma in situ, but we won't know until we do a biopsy."

Stunned. He'd said "it."

I flipped through the booklet to DCIS (ductal carcinoma in situ) while Steve asked questions. The two men spoke, their voices fading into the background as I read.

Now, the description of DCIS is pretty tame. It's considered pre-cancer when it's caught early. The minute the DCIS spills outside of the duct, it's considered invasive, and that's when things get complicated.

"I've seen a lot of DCIS," he said. "We won't know for sure it *is* DCIS until we explore. Now, we have a few options. We can do a needle biopsy or a wire guided surgical biopsy…"

Dr. Ruiz talked. Steve and I listened. But I felt as if I were having an out-of-body experience, almost as if the conversation was about someone else, as he expected us to make a decision on what kind of biopsy I'd like to have, as if we really *knew* anything about anything.

My thoughts went to the dark side. *But I have a two year old. How can he grow up without a mother?* This was the thought that kept bashing me over the head like a rock hammer. It alternated with this thought: *How do I know what kind of biopsy I'd like to have, right here on the spot?*

Steve asked him, simply, "What would you do?"

"I can't make the decision for you. I can only give you the information," Dr. Ruiz said in his flat, unemotional tone that was quickly becoming annoying. "You don't have to decide today. Take some time and think about it."

My dogged husband persisted.

"Okay. Well, what would you do if it were *your* wife?"

Steve is pretty tricky that way.

Dr. Ruiz, stoic and calm, knitted his brow, pursed his mouth, and said, "If it were my wife, I'd have the surgical biopsy."

Of course, Steve asked why*.

Dr. Ruiz explained that, if possible, once inside, he might be able to remove the mass. If he could get in there and really look at it, see what was actually in there, it could preclude the need for a second surgery.

So that's what I decided to do.

My surgical biopsy, under local anesthesia, was scheduled for the middle of December.

*[Tip: *This is a good example of why it's so important to have an advocate with you—an observer, another ear—for any kind of important medical decisions. Don't go by yourself, if you can help it. Sometimes it's hard to process all the information that is thrown at you during an especially stressful time.*

It's also a good idea to have a notebook or tablet with you to write down little notes to yourself.]

Let Me Get This Off My Chest

It's [Not] Funny When You Wake Up In The Middle Of Surgery

Humor is everywhere, in that there's irony in just about anything a human does.

~ *Bill Nye*

Before my surgical biopsy, I underwent the guided wire part of the procedure in which I basically had my breast squeezed again, just as if I were having a mammogram.

First, the technician inserted, very carefully, a wire into the tumor so that the surgeons would know exactly where to cut. It was a rather exacting procedure, and uncomfortable since Lefty was in the vise. After the wire had been inserted, the technician put a simple Styrofoam cup over the end where it stuck out of my breast.

I was wheeled into the surgery room and put under a strong local anesthesia. Sometime later, I woke on the operating table to this burning, tugging, sawing sensation. I was semiconscious. I knew I had pain, but the meds made it so that I didn't care. I lay there on the operating table and listened to the surgeon and his assisting surgeon talking to each other.

They noticed me stirring.

"Hey, it looks like someone's awake," the assisting surgeon said.

I mumbled something, probably nonsensical, like, "The blue banana lives under my front porch." Everything felt as if it were happening far away, in my la-la-land of drug haze. Then I said something like, "I've been listening to you."

The assisting surgeon tested me. "So, what have we been saying?"

"I kept hearing you say 'Kelly' and 'Kelly clamp.'"

For some reason—probably the drugs—I felt giddy. In the midst of my operation, I sensed there was something wrong with my wakeful state. This was *not* how it was supposed to be.

The surgeons remarked about my toughness and then said something like, "Why don't we give you a little something to put you back to sleep."

There was no argument from me.

In the recovery area, I threw up once, right into a small trash can that Steve grabbed quickly when I announced: "I'm going to throw up now."

Then I threw up again on the way home to my mother-in-law's to pick up Andrew.

Three days later, I got the bad news.

Steve sat with me in the exam room at Kaiser, and we listened as Dr. Ruiz gave the results: ductal carcinoma in situ that had become invasive.

"And I didn't get clear margins," he told us soberly.

Cancer is serious business, and Dr. Ruiz was a breast specialist. But, really, it wouldn't have hurt him to smile a little. Just a little. A crack. A hair. Something to let me know that it wasn't time to plan my funeral yet. His bed-side manner had room for improvement.

"Now, we can either do what's called breast conservation surgery or a mastectomy," he began.

The word "mastectomy" was like this flashing red sign in my head, hypnotizing me.

No, no, no. Not that.

"I'd rather have a lumpectomy," I said, finding my voice, absolutely confident in my decision.

We'd done our research, Steve and I. We'd read, and then read some more, especially since everybody and their mother had given us books about breasts, breast cancer, and everything known to womankind about breasts—I even had two copies of *Dr. Susan Love's Breast Book**. We knew the stats on recurrence after a lumpectomy combined with radiation and Tamoxifen.

Yeah, we were *that* good.

"Lumpectomy is certainly an option, but if I go in and don't get clean margins, I'll have to go back in again, and there's only so many times I can do that," he said, giving us full disclosure.

There was only so much breast to cut. I got it.

Steve went there again.

"What would you do if it were your wife?"

Dr. Ruiz gave a little sigh and in his calm way acknowledged, "If it were my wife, I'd probably advise a lumpectomy." He continued with his reasoning: "You can always have the mastectomy later, if there's a recurrence down the road."

In our, admittedly limited, research and non-medical backgrounds, we'd found that cancer involved a lot of percentages and statistics. Basically, statistically, the lowest chance of recurrence would have been for me to go with mastectomy followed by chemo if there were nodes involved—meaning the cancer had spread to the body's lymph nodes. If no nodes were involved, then maybe the mastectomy would be all that was needed.

If I opted for breast conservation, though, or lumpectomy, I'd need radiation, five years of Tamoxifen, and chemotherapy depending on the size of tumor and any nodal involvement.

I wasn't ready to give up my breast. I was so young— at least, that's what every one of the medical professionals had said. It was a common comment: "But you're so *young* for breast cancer."

Lucky me?

"I'll be happy with whatever there is left," I said.

I meant it. Whatever was left.

Let Me Get This Off My Chest

My lumpectomy surgery was scheduled for December 30th. Dr. Ruiz would attempt to remove the rest of the tumor, aiming for clear margins, but the tumor was a comedo type, which meant it was aggressive, and it was located close to the chest wall, which also complicated matters. In addition to the lumpectomy, I'd also have an axillary (under the arm) lymph node dissection at the same time to check for spreading of the cancer.

It was set.

Christmas was coming up. Our little family, we were trying to build traditions, and we *had* to keep going, keep putting one foot in front of the other, for our little boy.

So on the same day we scheduled my tumor removal and lymph node dissection, we drove to Target to pick out a Christmas tree.

In bed that night, as the reality of my situation came crashing in, Steve held me as I sobbed, letting myself go for the first time. My tears fell on his shoulders as he became my sanctuary.

Life was feeling all too real.

[**Tip:** It's never a bad idea to get a second opinion. After my surgical biopsy, I arranged to have a copy of my pathology report and slides read by a pathologist at another medical institution to see if that pathologist concurred with the findings of the Kaiser pathologist, which he did.

Ask your doctor about getting a second opinion. It won't offend them; they're used to it. If it does, you may have the wrong doctor. Your medical care is your care.

Dr. Susan Love's Breast Book is now in its sixth edition and is a comprehensive guide and resource about breast cancer.]

People Gave Me Books, *Not* Donuts

**Donuts.
Is there
anything they
can't do?**

~ Homer Simpson

After word got out about my diagnosis, I started hearing from people out of the blue. First came a call from a woman who was part of a local program called Breast Buddies. She shared her story with me, eager to talk, describing her double mastectomy. She'd had two rounds of chemo but elected to stop—it had made her very ill—opting for herbal remedies instead. As she told her story, I listened, and it was almost as if I had been placed in a support role for her. It was a little overwhelming. One thing she emphasized was the importance of washing fruits and vegetables while undergoing chemotherapy as a means of staying healthy, and she made me promise to buy veggie wash. I promised.

A week or so later, I went to a health food store and bought a bottle. I used it once to wash our bag of apples, and it made me feel like a good mother. Really virtuous! Then I put it under the sink and forgot about it. (In my defense, I had a lot of other things to think about. Plus, I'm lazy.)

Next was a call from a woman who knew my mother-in-law. She'd had breast cancer fifty years prior, undergoing a mastectomy back in the days when the doctors took more of the breast and surrounding tissue than they needed to. Her call comforted me since she was, and is, still here all these years later.

Besides hearing from people who'd had breast cancer, I also received a mountain of information about breast cancer. Everyone wanted to contribute. I will admit, though, receiving two copies of *Dr. Susan Love's Breast Book* wasn't as exciting as seeing a box of donuts magically appear on my front porch mat, but the books helped me in my continuing education, and I was able to give the extra copy to someone else.

I was given a funny book about breast cancer, I was given serious books, and the coordinator from Kaiser gave me a bag full of dry educational pamphlets with lots of clip art diagrams of breasts.

It was all a bit of information overload. I read through the books until I couldn't read any more, then put them in a pile next to my bed. When I'd had enough, I moved the pile of books to the bookcase in the den, then later out to the garage where the ones that hadn't been given away remain to this day.

I knew I had breast cancer and wanted the cancer removed; what I didn't need was the constant reminder of the disease.

Bargaining With God

**Before God
we are all
equally wise –
and equally
foolish.**
~ *Albert Einstein*

When I first received my cancer diagnosis, my thoughts leapt to my son, crashing and colliding into each other in my brain. Andrew, at two years old, was a generally happy little guy, and we were so very close, as moms and their sons usually are. His hair was long and blond with bowl-cut bangs (unprofessionally sculpted by yours truly when they'd grow too long over his eyes and my mother-in-law threatened to give him braids). He was my buddy.

I needed some extra insurance.

First, my bargaining with God went like this:

Dear God, please let me be there for Andrew while he's growing up.

My own father had passed away suddenly, unexpectedly, when I was thirteen, leaving me devastated. It's a terrible thing to lose a parent at any age, but while still growing up—it's too much. Too cruel. So I began pestering God pretty much all day long, figuring if one prayer weren't enough, He *couldn't* ignore them if they were offered up on the half hour.

Soon my bargaining with God went like this:

Dear God, please let me be there for Andrew when he graduates high school.

Then my bargaining with God went like this:

Dear God, please let me be there for Andrew's wedding; please let me see him marry a good woman. Someone who really deserves him. (A universal mother's prayer.)

Then my bargaining went like this:

Dear God, please let me be there to see my first grandchild.

Then my bargaining went like this:

Dear God, please let me meet my grandchildren.

See what I did there? I lengthened my supplications. While my first prayer would only get me to age eighteen, my last prayer—if he waited and married in his late twenties and had kids a year or two or three after—well, then I'd bought myself some real time.

I say this a little in jest, but I've prayed all along. If nothing else, God has been my sounding board and companion. He probably shakes his head, laughing at me, but that's okay, because it means He hears me.

All I can say is: so far, so good.

What To Say To Someone With Breast Cancer

It sounds trite, but in relationships, you have to communicate.

~ *Peter Krause*

Sometimes it was the smallest things that kept my spirits up—a call, an email. Nothing big, except that the other person had paused, taking a moment or two out of their day to let me know they were thinking about me. Then there were people who should have said something but didn't. (I say "should have" because of the place they held in my life. Maybe they were a neighbor or I was related to them, but I'm not naming names here. And if you're reading this book, then it wasn't you.) Luckily, in my world of connections, there were only a few who remained silent.

Saying nothing is as bad as saying the completely wrong thing. People don't always know what to say when someone has had something really crappy happen to them, so they don't say anything at all, leaving the person grappling with their bad news or sudden loss feeling as if the silent friend or relative doesn't care. This is not a good feeling.

We need acknowledgment. We need someone to say: "I recognize what you're going through, and I'm here for you." That is all.

So my all-purpose advice when a loved one receives an upsetting diagnosis or has faced the loss of someone dear to them: at the very least, send a card.

Keep it simple and speak from the heart. Don't tell them you know what they're going through, or that it's all for the best, or it's part of God's plan, because they may end up wanting to hurt you.

What to say? Feel free to choose from the following list. (Or mix and match, if you're feeling extra bold.)

1. I am so sorry, and I just wanted you to know that you're in my thoughts. Add "prayers" if this person is religious and would appreciate prayers. Don't say you'll pray unless you mean it.

2. Let me know if there's anything I can do for you.

3. I'm here for you if you need to talk.

4. Would you like to get out of the house and get some coffee?

5. Do you need me to pick up anything from the store?

After I'd received the bad news from my doctor, and once my lumpectomy surgery was scheduled, my friend Katie came bearing See's candies, and we sat at my kitchen table with the box of chocolates between us. I talked a little about what was going on and told her about my upcoming surgery, but mainly I sat and listened to Katie's funny stories about the different people (mostly ex-boyfriends) in her life and watched her mimic them with impersonations and hand gestures.

In the midst of the most chaotic stream of emotions I felt about my upcoming surgery, life, death, and everything, I sat and laughed with my old friend, wiping tears away. Good, happy tears. She didn't try to tell me it was all for the best; she didn't give me any advice. She was just there as my friend, taking my mind off my problems for a little while. It was the best thing anyone could have done for me at that time, and even though that was thirteen years ago, it stands out in my memory, and I'll never forget her kindness (even if she's long since forgotten it).

Bottom line: don't remain silent. And if you really can't think of the right thing to say, send chocolate.

Hangin' With Father John

Every moment and every event of every man's life on earth plants something in his soul.

~ *Thomas Merton*

The morning of my lumpectomy, I was fighting a bad cough. I'd been warned that illness of any type could cause my surgery to be postponed, and I'd caught a cold that had gone into my chest the week before. Of course. It was my Annual Christmas Cold.

Now, the last thing a person who's made their mind up about surgery wants is to have their surgery pushed back. But it was one of those rumbly coughs. I lay there in the pre-op area, on my bed, trying to will myself not to cough, *trying* to suppress the urge.

"You'd better let them know," Steve urged.

"I don't want them to cancel my surgery," I protested.

"If you cough during the operation, it might cause them to screw up."

Now, that was a terrible, terrifying, horrific thought.

When the anesthesiologist stopped by to introduce himself, I fessed up and told him I had a cold. He looked at me without concern, took out his stethoscope, listened to my chest and nodded. He didn't seem to care.

Steve shrugged his shoulders. At least we were comforted to know my coughing wouldn't cause an unfortunate scalpel accident.

My steady rock of a husband sat next to me and held my hand, willing me to be strong. We still had an hour and a half to kill before the scheduled start time, when to my not-so-pleasant surprise, my mother-in-law's priest came striding up to be with us.

It sounds mean, but I wasn't thrilled to see Father John. Dressed in his black clericals, macrame belt, Birkenstocks, black socks, with a large Celtic cross hanging from his neck, his look was casual clergy.

The terrible part is that I guess I wanted to wait in silent misery with the man I loved. Father John was not going to permit that. There would be no silent misery. Not that day.

"How are you, Margaret?" He asked simply, with sincere compassion. My reservations about having him there melted away when he told us about how my mother-in-law Sue—steady, pragmatic, not one for flights of fancy or casual acts of spontaneity—walked up to him before service one Sunday and handed him a note while tears streamed down her face.

She couldn't speak the words to tell him that I had breast cancer.

If I ever think bad thoughts about my mother-in-law (which I never, ever do) all I have to do is picture this scene.

I will never forget Father John's act of kindness. Steve and I didn't even attend his church. It was, like, a twenty-minute drive, and we were serious Sunday morning slackers.

He cared anyway though, even though we'd had the most minimal of contact, maybe meeting a handful of times since he'd taken over as priest. He was a good man; a true man of God. It showed on his face, his countenance, his touch, the way he put his hand on my shoulder and grasped my hand in his.

We chatted the time away. He asked about my life with Steve and Andrew, and I managed somehow to feel calmed by his presence. It ended up being a really *good* thing to have his counsel in the minutes before surgery.

As the attendant came to wheel my bed away, Father John stopped, held my hand and Steve's hand, and asked God to watch over me and to guide the surgeons and nurses.

I drifted off, and Steve told me later that Father John stayed with my group in the waiting room trading stories, laughing, and counseling my mother whose worry level was at maximum. He remained to have lunch with them at the Kaiser cafeteria, and he was still waiting with them when Dr. Ruiz came out of surgery, dressed in his scrubs looking triumphant, clenching his fist, making that little "Yes!" move.

Dr. Ruiz seemed confident he'd gotten it all and just couldn't help himself. In that moment he was Superman after saving Lois Lane.

Things were looking up.

That night, after throwing up in recovery from the anesthesia, and after throwing up again at home, Steve put me to bed with pain medication.

The next night was New Year's Eve. I mostly stayed in bed, in pain from the lumpectomy, but in even more pain from the axillary dissection. I lay there, listening to the voices of my mother, my sisters, and my nieces.

My family had come over to celebrate New Year's Eve, even though I couldn't really join them. I did venture out for a few minutes but had to creep back to bed—there was too much throbbing, pulsing pain, pulling and tugging. It felt like I was overdoing it a little.

But I lay there listening to the laughter, the voices, and felt the love emanating from the next room, like this little bubble of warmth enveloping me. My mom was worried about me—her daughter with breast cancer—and I thought about how unfair that part of it was—not for me, but for her.

I thought of my mom, how much she loved me, and cried.

Animals In Wigs

**Beauty in
things exists
in the mind which
contemplates them.**
~ *David Hume*

On January 2nd, three days after my surgery, I got the call from Dr. Ruiz letting me know he had clear margins. Beneath his veneer of calmness, I *thought* I detected a hint of happiness in his voice. Just a hint.

Good news. Fantastic news. The cancer had been removed. Gone. And even better news: the lymph nodes were clear.

Steve and I celebrated and started calling people to tell them the good news.

A post-op appointment with Dr. Ruiz was scheduled to determine my next step.

Let Me Get This Off My Chest

My tumor, the invasive portion, was small, half a centimeter, which, according to the National Cancer Institute's* guidelines, was staged at a IA, the lowest on a scale of I to IV.

Dr. Ruiz remained confident I'd undergo chemotherapy, even though the NCI guidelines did *not* indicate that chemo was necessary. (Steve and I had been doing our research online.)

Dr. Ruiz was the surgeon, though, not the medical oncologist** whom I'd be meeting with in two weeks to determine my follow-up treatment.

In the meantime, Steve went online and ordered a wig. Apparently in my husband's fantasy world, I am a redhead.

Somehow when I wasn't looking, Steve put together a pre-chemotherapy party so we could get together with friends and family and have a celebration before I'd start chemotherapy, get sick, feel terrible, and lose my hair.

Gifts were brought, good times with friends and family were had. Many hugs were exchanged.

And then there was "the wig."

Perhaps because of the alcohol, or maybe just due to a party's natural evolution, every person in attendance had their picture taken wearing the bright maroon/fuchsia wig. My sisters wore the wig; my brother-in-law wore the wig: our Australian Shepherd wore the wig; both cats wore the wig...

Surprisingly, the person who looked best wearing the wig was our friend Bruce. He made a very good-looking woman, even if he did look like an Amsterdam hooker.

*[*The National Cancer Institute is part of the National Institutes of Health. It is the recognized authority on cancer staging and is a very good resource for information on all types of cancer.*

**Most people will see different doctors for their treatment. My surgical oncologist was responsible for my treatment during the biopsy and surgery phase, while my treatment post-surgery was overseen by a medical oncologist who determined my care and treatment from that point forward.]*

My Support Group Experience

We sail within a vast sphere, ever drifting in uncertainty, driven from end to end.
~ *Blaise Pascal*

One day, I got a call out of the blue from my husband's cousin Sherry whom I'd met only a handful of times. As fate would have it, she'd been diagnosed with a different form of breast cancer right around the same time that I had been. Her stage was higher than mine—either a IIB or IIIA, her doctors weren't quite sure which—and she would be undergoing chemotherapy soon.

Sherry was seven years older, liked to joke around, and was very enthusiastic, talking fast with a lot to say. She called several times, came over to my house and visited, and we quickly bonded over our shared experience.

She found a breast cancer support group and invited me to go with her.

What I found out about the support group was that there are many different kinds of breast cancer patients. Some women were stage I like me, some were stage IV with metastasis, some had lumpectomies with radiation, some had mastectomies with chemotherapy. In the room of women, breast cancer took many forms.

We listened to a young woman in ripped jeans with a red bandanna over her bald head as she told her heartfelt story, describing how her brothers and sisters kept a vase of fresh flowers on her dresser in her bedroom. They'd refill the vase every few days, so she'd always have something beautiful to look at as she lay in bed, sick from the chemo. What struck me about her was her age; she was no more than twenty.

A woman in her forties, stage IV, spoke about how her doctor had recently found a small spot on her lung and was planning to biopsy it. She was stoic and matter-of-fact about things. She didn't dissolve into an emotional mess but remained calm, planning to face her future head-on. I felt tears coming to the surface as she spoke about her kids in elementary and middle school, and her supportive husband.

It was almost too much to deal with, but the support the women had for each other was unmistakably there.

When it was my turn around the table, I told my story—lumpectomy, stage IA, DCIS with a half-centimeter invasive portion, no nodes—and I felt guilty, as if mine wasn't serious enough by comparison. Then I felt dumb for feeling guilty. The inner voices in my head fought; I couldn't shut them up. (This happens to me a lot.)

Sherry and I talked about the group on the way home. She'd found it too depressing, too much reality hitting her in the face all at once. I had mixed emotions, and when I think about it now, I think it was too early in the process for me and may have been better down the road a few weeks or months later as I dealt with getting back to "normal" life (whatever that means).

We decided not to go back.

[**Tip:** *People will share their individual stories with you. Keep in mind that their experience may not necessarily be anything like yours. Each case is different. Still, it helps to talk with people who understand what you're going through.*]

Life Lessons Are Ongoing

You have succeeded in life when all you really want is only what you really need.
~ *Vernon Howard*

There is no way a person can undergo cancer without learning a few life lessons.

Where do I go from here?

What will I take away from this experience?

There's got to be some sort of silver lining; right?

One thing was certain for me: I wouldn't ever go back to being a person who *hadn't* gotten a cancer diagnosis. It was now an irrefutable part of me, just like the fact that I was a woman, a court reporter, a mother, a wife, a sister. I would now add breast cancer survivor to the list of things I was; I am.

What did I learn in the first few weeks as my newly diagnosed breast cancer survivor self? Perhaps the most important life lesson: cancer, in a way, had pretty quickly pulled my life into sharp focus, bringing with it a new perspective. I knew who the most important people were—my family and my close friends, the ones who would have my back when I really needed them.

I no longer wanted to waste time around negative people or energy-sucking vampires, those types who would make me feel inadequate or bad about myself. It's not that I was going to actively go out of my way to X people out of my life; I wasn't going to call them up and say, "Hey, you suck. You're out." I just wasn't going to worry about them anymore. Or really try not to, at the very least.

And I learned to say no, which is something women especially have a hard time with—we don't want to disappoint anyone. But there are always, it seems, people out there with requests for our time. Sometimes it's okay to turn things down or maybe be a bit more selective about commitments we accept. And is there *really* anything wrong with buying store-bought cupcakes for your kid's classroom event? It's okay. We don't *all* need to be Martha Stewart.

Would I use my breast cancer patient/survivor status to occasionally weasel out of things I didn't want to do? Damn straight! But I also felt the weight of the years ahead of me—hopefully—that necessitated that I take care of myself, manage my stress load, and not work too hard. I wanted to be a little kinder to myself so that, hopefully, my cancer wouldn't return. (I mean, if I had any kind of control over it returning.)

My profession, court reporting, is a very physical, tough job. It's enough to make a person crazy at times, and working with Type A personalities on multi-million-dollar cases can be extremely stressful. Long days of pounding on the steno machine would leave me with sore arms and wrists. Often, I'd feel stress in my neck and gut when the parties would argue and attorneys would make demands. I knew I'd have to manage my workload to minimize stress and help my overall health. From that time on, I made it a priority to accept fewer work assignments.

That leads me to another life lesson: getting by with less.

There's a line from the Steely Dan song *Reelin' In the Years* that I think about a lot when I'm considering mate-rial things and what I really need versus what I want.

Donald Fagen sings the line about how we often don't recognize what is right in front of our face, or that which we hold in our hands, as precious and meaningful. We keep reaching for something else.

I think about this when I see people working so hard, running on that never-ending treadmill, to pay for things they covet, as if that thing will bring them inner peace, happiness, and will be the key to [*fill in the blank*]. I tried to focus more on the things that were precious and less on the extraneous.

Life is short, and no one on their death bed has ever regretted *not* spending more time at work. Since I decided to work less, I got used to having less and learned fairly quickly that I didn't need as much as I thought. (Don't the organizational experts say we only wear twenty percent of what's in our closet anyway? Okay, I made up that number right now, but it's something like that.)

I strove to take the lessons learned from cancer with me into my daily life; I didn't want to forget and start taking things for granted.

So I guess maybe what I'm trying to say is this: when life gives you crap, if possible, make lemonade. Or something like that.

Playing The Cancer Card

Sometimes the only way to deal with horrific things in life is through a dark sense of humor.
~ *Margaret Cho*

I'm not necessarily saying you *should* play the cancer card, but when going through something so crappy, there should be a little perk here and there, shouldn't there?

Steve accused me of playing the cancer card only once. When I was sure I was about to start chemotherapy any day (according to the information my surgeon had given me), and just before the chemotherapy party with the fantasy wig, I called my hairdresser Michael.

"Is there any way you can fit me in?" I asked, in my sweetest angel voice.

"I'm completely booked today, but I can see you in two weeks from now, if you want a Saturday appointment."

"Oh," I said, disappointed. "It's just that I'm going to be starting chemotherapy in a week or so and I was hoping I could get in for a haircut. You know, so it doesn't all fall out in long chunks."

I could hear him flipping his book.

"How about Tuesday morning? Can you come in at nine?"

Steve heard our conversation and was not about to let me get away with it—he's very good about calling me on things, Mr. Judgmental One.

"I can't believe you just played the cancer card," he said, half joking, half accusing when I got off the phone.

"I *didn't*!"

Okay. He was right. But I wasn't sorry then; I'm not sorry now.

I repeat: if you're going through something as crappy as cancer and little, nice things can happen to you, like maybe getting that good table in the restaurant, "Because I have cancer," (and cough a couple of times, looking tragic) or moving up to the front of the movie line, "Because I have cancer and I can't stand around too long, my ankles start to swell," said with a sweet smile— the littlest things like that—how can that be wrong?

[**Tip and a warning:** *Play the cancer card wisely, though, or else your friends and family will catch on to your tricks, and you'll have to go to the back of the line with all the humdrum non-cancer people.]*

Second Opinions, And An Exit

Never go to a doctor whose office plants have died.

~ *Erma Bombeck*

After my lumpectomy and axillary dissection, when I met with Dr. Linda Rossi, my medical oncologist, she let me know that my stage IA cancer with no nodes indicated no chemotherapy was warranted.

"Really? Are you sure? Dr. Ruiz said I'd have chemotherapy."

She gave me this look like: "Are you kidding me?" Then said, "You don't need it. Why have it when you don't need it?"

This threw me for a loop, but in a good way. The best of all possible ways.

That's when I called Sherry, my husband's cousin, to let her know I wouldn't be having chemo as planned.

"Are you sure? Don't you think it's a mistake? What if it comes back? I mean, I know I don't want *mine* coming back."

Her words stung. Did she think I wanted mine to return?

I stifled my hurt response, awkwardly assuring her I wasn't making a mistake. She remained steadfast, urging me to reconsider my oncologist's advice, and I promised to call her back after getting a second opinion.

She was only doing this because she was worried about my health.

After my lumpectomy, I had not one, but two medical oncologists. Besides Dr. Rossi—who would oversee any additional therapy, including drug therapy, and would, as she'd told me, follow up with me *for the rest of my life*— I'd been assigned a radiation oncologist, Dr. Chu.

Dr. Chu looked as if he'd just graduated high school—energetic and enthusiastic. He was small of stature, slim, and a little on the bouncy side. When we first met, he shook my hand and looked into my eyes and told me, "You're going to be fine. IA? No problem," brushing my cancer away. "We'll just radiate you as protection. It's an insurance policy."

I *really* loved his confidence.

Dr. Chu was part of the Hollywood Kaiser system. He concurred with Dr. Rossi, agreeing that I didn't need chemotherapy but suggested that I could get an additional opinion with the Kaiser Hollywood oncology board.

So that's exactly what I did. Steve and I spoke to the head oncologist in Hollywood who then took my case before the cancer review board where they discussed it and agreed: Dr. Rossi was right; no chemo.

When I called Sherry to let her know I'd gotten a second (and third) opinion, I spoke to her husband.

"So, I heard you got some good news."

It was funny because he didn't sound happy at all; he sounded pissed. Probably pissed that his wife would be going through the ugly thing, and I wouldn't. It was as if I'd broken a contract or something.

That's when Sherry cut me out of her life, and I realized that how each individual reacts to cancer is not the same.

Sometimes we cling to people going through a similar experience out of a need for solidarity or comfort. For a few weeks, Sherry and I shared a similar experience. That is, until she found out I wouldn't be going through chemotherapy. Then, she dropped me.

It wasn't a good feeling.

A few phone calls, a gift bag left on her doorstep, and a card sent on my end; nothing back on hers.

I didn't have to have chemo, my invasive portion was small; it was caught earlier than hers.

In the months to come, she would have a bone marrow transplant, would spend time in isolation, enduring pain and sickness that I'll never know, and I'd betrayed her by not sharing the experience.

We haven't spoken since, but I did see her a few months ago at a cafeteria. She looked good, but older, as I'm sure I do too. We smiled at each other, and it was one of those things where I didn't realize who she was until the moment had passed, making it too late to say anything.

I wish her well.

Radiation And Tiny Tattoos

Life isn't a matter of milestones, but of moments.

~ *Rose Kennedy*

Since I'd opted for a lumpectomy and not a mastectomy, my treatment included radiation therapy. Five days a week for six consecutive weeks, Steve and I made the trip into Hollywood to Kaiser's radiation facility, with its state-of-the-art equipment. (The Kaiser facility, sadly, is nowhere near the "fun" Hollywood tourist attractions. The area is fairly nondescript with mostly office buildings and parking structures.)

After first undergoing a PET-CT scan and my exact tumor location—or former tumor location, since it had been removed—had been mapped, I was tattooed by one of the technicians, which was another new experience for me. What it felt like was someone poking a latch hook into my chest. Six times. It was painful but over quickly. (For someone who's had actual tattoos placed on their body, this would be no big deal. Keep in mind, I'm kind of a baby about things.) The marker tattoos are permanent and make me feel like I'm part of the "in crowd." (Not really.)

"Does radiation hurt?"

That is probably the most common question I've been asked over the years about radiation therapy, and I can only answer from the perspective of a breast cancer patient, since the side effects of radiation vary depending on the location of the body and the type of cancer.

In my experience, no, it didn't hurt. The actual radiation treatments were painless. The only pain involved was comparable to having a slight sunburn after the daily dose of directed radiation had built up and burned the skin. By the fifth week, I developed a burn where the underside of the breast rested against the chest and the skin wasn't able to air out. Initially, it started out as bubbles or blisters that hurt a little and needed special topical cream*, which I applied for the last two weeks of treatment. It worked surprisingly well, and the skin was much better in just a few days.

My radiation appointments were at the same time each day, 1:10 p.m., and once I checked in at the desk and my number was called, things moved rapidly. I'd change into a gown from the waist up and then be taken into the room containing the radiation accelerator. The tech would have me lie down on the table, dial the precise location in, move the machine into the exact right place, then leave the room to administer the dose. This whole process would take about fifteen minutes each day.

Steve and I would drop Andrew off at my mother-in-law's house on our way in to Hollywood. Almost each day, when we'd return to pick him up, we'd find the two of them sitting on her driveway with fat sticks of sidewalk chalk in their hands, drawing pictures of the planets, of dogs, flowers, bees, and other things, using the whole driveway as their palette. Sometimes my mother-in-law Sue would have Andrew lie on the ground, and she'd trace his body with the chalk, so there would be a chalk outline of our boy. But it wasn't in a creepy CSI crime scene drawing sort of way. It was sweet; our little boy growing up.

One thing that stood out about my radiation experience was the staff. The technicians were mostly young, in their twenties, friendly, supportive, and professional. The two on my last day—a young woman and young man—hugged me after my treatment. We'd bonded over the short time. They saw me as a person and recognized my existence; I wasn't just one more in an endless line of patients. I'll always remember their compassion, given at a time when I sorely needed it, and how something as small as a touch can create a connection with someone.

Another memory I have is of a little boy at the radiation facility who was slightly older than Andrew. He received radiation treatments at the same time that I did. Each day I'd see him, this boy with a bald head who acted like a typical three year old. His parents read to him, keeping him occupied until his number was called, never showing any outward sign of the complicated emotions they must have been feeling. Each day I saw him, my heart hurt a little, and I thought about my own little boy and the randomness of cancer.

Seeing him was a daily lesson in perspective; I had so much to be grateful for in my own life.

Daily naps. Being a self-admitted, lifelong napper, a natural after-radiation practice was for me to come home and nap for an hour, sometimes two.

Some people say radiation makes a person tired. My naps were more, I think, a coping mechanism, though; a little rest of the body and brain. I needed the decompression time. Whether I was actually physically tired, I'm not sure. It just felt right.

Before I knew it, the six weeks were over. The time passed quickly, believe it or not, and by the end, I was ready to go back to work, to get on with my life.

Or at least I tried to convince myself that I was ready to get on with my life.

[*Biafine is a topical non-steroidal cream used to treat burns and wounds and is often used in conjunction with radiation treatment. I was given several packets of Biafine from the radiation technicians.]

Moving On, Internal Pep Talks

Strength is the capacity to break a chocolate bar into four pieces with your bare hands— and then eat just one of the pieces.

~ *Judith Viorst*

During the period of my lumpectomy and radiation back in 1999-2000, I was off work for approximately four months. What I found during that time was that the physical recovery was maybe half; the other half was mental. I had to overcome my fear of moving on. Really, there were a multitude of fears—the fear of going back into the world, of having this invisible sign hanging around my neck that read: "This person had breast cancer."

I felt like part of my journey up the mountain of recovery was dealing with the fact that my life had changed; I had this cancer experience that was an inextricable part of me, something in my psyche, imbedded in my being.

Returning to work, for some reason, felt scary. Attorneys I'd known for years had no idea what I'd been through. It felt odd, almost like I was hiding this big secret. (A big secret that had absolutely no effect on the way I was able to perform my job, but somehow, I just *felt* different.)

Something I learned quickly upon returning to work: survivors are everywhere.

One of my first assignments after going back was an employment hearing for the Immigration and Naturalization Service headquartered in Downtown Los Angeles. The hearing took place in their own version of a courtroom, before a judge, with attorneys for the plaintiff and defendant. It was a three-day job, and I'd overheard one of the expert witnesses for the plaintiff talking about how he'd been on leave for prostate cancer treatment.

During a break, I went over and chatted with him, sharing that I'd been off work for my own cancer treatment. It was the first time I'd confided to anyone publicly about my experience, and the feeling of vulnerability was as if I'd taken off my shirt and shown him my scars. The man's demeanor changed instantly; we were part of "the club"—the club no one wants to be a member of. We swapped stories, and I watched him choke up while telling me about his journey.

Here was this complete stranger opening up to me, telling me how glad he was to be alive, and how his family and grandchildren meant everything to him; the cancer had put his priorities in place.

So it wasn't just *me* who'd been given the gift of clarity and perspective.

On the last day of the hearing, I packed my equipment up and walked out to the parking structure with the judge, a younger African-American woman, maybe twenty-eight or twenty-nine. In the midst of a hot flash, I joked about it, fanning myself with my hand. She gave me a funny look, and I explained that I was taking Tamoxifen, which causes hot flashes. As we walked, she opened up to me, telling me about her recent mastectomy, gesturing to her wig.

We stopped and chatted for a little while before she had to run off and meet friends for dinner. We hugged; strangers no more.

Survivors are everywhere.

Tamoxifen:
Oh, Joy!
(Not Really)

It's too hot.
~ The Author

After a breast cancer diagnosis, after surgery, chemo-therapy, and/or radiation, most women are prescribed medication to prevent recurrence. This is complex—a-gain, where the medical oncologist will figure in—and depends on many things, such as a woman's pre-menopause or post-menopause status, since different medications are used depending upon which group she falls into, and whether her cancer type is estrogen recep-tor positive or estrogen receptor negative, et cetera.

Since I was pre-menopausal by quite a few years, and because my tumor was estrogen receptor positive, I was prescribed Tamoxifen, ten milligrams, twice daily.

For the first time in my life, I found myself using a pill keeper. But pill keepers are for old people; right? I mean, don't you have to have a membership in AARP to use one?

I felt *so* like my grandmother. But I'd never been good with pills. Medication and I have never gotten along, for some reason. It does weird things to me. My chi is wrong or something, I don't know. During the short period of time I was on birth control pills, I'd often forget my pill and then have to take two.

A pill keeper was now part of my daily life.

Dr. Rossi warned me, "It might send you into a pre-menopausal state."

"Huh? What does that mean?"

"Well, you might have some hot flashes. You may go through something that mimics menopause, but it shouldn't last."

"How *long* will it last?"

She laughed. "I don't know. A few months maybe? Everyone's different."

"What can I take for the hot flashes?"

Since breast cancers can be fueled by estrogen, there was no way I could take anything that messed with my hormones.

"Soy is supposed to be good for the hot flashes," she said, then shrugged. I could tell she was reaching with the soy; I was on my own.

So at the age of thirty-four, I found myself plunging into hot flashes at the drop of a hat. Just thinking about my body's internal temperature would cause my face to flush. My forehead would break out into little dots of perspiration, and at night—every night—I'd throw the covers off, even though it was March and cool at night, and Steve would be left shivering, comforter-less.

Poor Steve.

The up side is that after about six months, my Tamoxifen hot flashes subsided; my body had gotten used to it. I went along with my life.

At the end of five years, Steve got out his video camera and took a film of me. First I gave a little speech—which I've since forgotten—then I deposited my Tamoxifen bottles into the trash.

Five years of Tamoxifen marked five years post my breast cancer diagnosis, during which time I'd been seen by Dr. Rossi at least twice a year, receiving a full blood work-up before each appointment. Dr. Rossi would go over the blood test results, including those tests looking for cancer markers, and she'd do a physical exam, probing my breasts for lumps or changes to the tissue. I also had mammograms, which, after the first year, were knocked down from twice to once a year. My radiation oncologist, Dr. Chu, stopped my visits after two years, declaring me cured, in his very enthusiastic manner.

At five years without recurrence, breast cancer was officially part of my past. So to help mark my five-year anniversary, Steve, Andrew, and I walked up together during church one Sunday morning, and our priest gave me a special blessing to mark my symbolic new beginning. We held hands and tears streamed down my face.

I said goodbye (mostly) to cancer.

*[**Tip:** To help with hot flashes, I found that a regular bandanna soaked with water and tied around my neck helped a lot when my body would randomly decide to stoke the furnace. If you're in bed when a hot flash kicks in, try putting a small towel on your pillow, and then tie the wet bandanna loosely at the neck. This also works for non-Tamoxifen-related hot flashes. Trust me.]*

Chugging Along With Lefty

- March 2012

Change is inevitable. Change is constant.

~ *Benjamin Disraeli*

Even though Lefty was a quarter smaller than Righty, she filled in my bras. We were *good* with each other. Solid. Things between us were copacetic.

In truth, Lefty was mostly for show. Ever since my lumpectomy, she remained tender, without much sensation in the nipple. Steve learned to handle her with extreme care or risk getting barked at. He had a healthy respect for Lefty (and my barkiness).

Over the next few years, Andrew grew and thrived; our lives were happy. Because of my medical history, we kept to our own one-child policy, but we were okay with it.

As with most people, along with the good, we suffered heartbreaking losses—first Steve's dad, then my brother Jon. We also felt the effects of the Great Recession economy through a lack of work, both of us being independent contractors. Mostly, though, we were happy. I'd taken the lessons and perspective gained from my first bout with breast cancer to heart, always at least *trying* to remember where I'd been and all that I had to be grateful for. And, really, there was always something to be thankful for, no matter how tenuous things became. As long as I kept to the basics, looked at the people in my life, those that were most precious to me, and didn't worry about the rest, I'd be fine. We'd be fine. The kitchen and bath remodel would have to wait. And wait. (Um, still waiting.)

As Steve would always remind me when I was in need of reassurance (in those times when he'd seek to talk me down from the verge of a meltdown) things would work out. And they usually did.

But I had to keep my mantra going: things don't matter; people do. We shopped thrift stores, mostly stopped eating out, gave thanks, and tried to keep an attitude of gratitude. Tried.

In March of 2012, at age forty-six, firmly entrenched in the whole midlife/menopause thing, I found out that my routine mammogram had revealed abnormal cells, and I knew Lefty and I would be no more; we'd soon be history.

I'd been warned that if there was a recurrence, mastectomy was the only option—no more cutting. Besides, my DCIS the second time was multi-focal; there was no way the different sections of it could be cut out and removed entirely.

Lefty and I would soon say goodbye.

Let Me Get This Off My Chest

Things Not To Say To A Person Facing Mastectomy

Better to remain silent and be thought a fool than to speak out and remove all doubt.

~ *Abraham Lincoln*

This: "Well, at least you get new boobs."

People want to put a positive light, the best possible spin, on a bad situation. It's human nature, I guess, to make crappy things seem less crappy. But when I told people about my upcoming mastectomy, a few said something lame.

For some reason, when the well-meaning people said things which resembled the aforementioned, I wanted to punch them in the face.

I didn't want new boobs.

I wasn't aiming for perfection.

I'm a jeans and tennies girl, I can swear like a sailor—especially when no one else is around—and I don't spend a lot of time on my hair. A sad little boobie was okay with me.

Not only did I have to get used to the idea of having a mastectomy, but I needed to decide what kind of re-construction. And this is where things get a little com-plicated.

The breast care coordinator I'd been referred to, after first talking to a very kind doctor who went over the re-sults of my biopsy, took out her book and showed me different women with their shirts off, modeling their re-constructed breasts. She presented three options for my consideration.

There was the DIEP flap procedure, which involved taking a large skin graft from the abdomen, forming new breasts, and injecting them with abdominal tissue (fat). This option sounded way too painful, although tempting.

(I'd get rid of unwanted belly fat, the kind that's very hard to lose once a person hits middle age. Bonus!)

Then there was the latissimus dorsi tissue flap procedure which involved creating a tunnel and cutting skin, fat, and muscle from the back and shoulder area and bringing it forward, still attached to the blood supply, to form the new breasts.

This also sounded painful.

The third option given to me—and the most appealing because of its simplicity and shorter hospital stay—was the placement of tissue expanders, or temporary implants, which would go in place of my old breasts. They'd be injected with saline over a period of weeks while the skin stretched, then the permanent implants would be exchanged at a later date.

I'd been warned, though, that since I'd previously received radiation to the breast, the scar tissue might not allow for the tissue expander procedure to work.

I processed this.

Steve's input—which I gave great weight to, since I trust him—was for me to go with the tissue expanders and get the smallest implants possible just to give me a little something on my chest and lessen the chance of complications.

I really wish I would have had the nerve to say, "Screw it. I don't need implants. I'm going to just go with the mastectomy. I'm going to be proud of my no-breast status."

I salute my sisters in the world who've gone this route. I wasn't quite brave enough.

After carefully thinking it over, I decided to go for reconstruction. I thought, psychologically, it would be easier to have something on my chest to look at that wouldn't be a reminder of cancer. Or at least *less* of a reminder.

[To learn more about breast reconstruction visit BreastReconstruction.org; a comprehensive resource for breast reconstruction: http://www.breastreconstruction.org/index.htm]

One Lump,
Or Two?

**The art of living is
more like wrestling
than dancing.**
~ *Marcus Aurelius*

Getting one's mind wrapped around a single mastectomy
is one thing; having your whole world rocked by the no-
tion of bilateral—having two breasts removed at once—is a whole different story. This is where my friend
Sally comes in.

Sally had undergone her own battle with breast cancer a few years earlier. I never knew what type of cancer
she had; I don't think *she* ever knew. She wasn't as con-
cerned with details—quite the opposite from me, a person who probably spends way too much time reading and

looking things up on the Internet, half of the time scaring myself. But Sally's was a larger tumor, she went through many rounds of chemotherapy, lost all of her hair, and her body was wracked and ravaged. Sally went through quite a bit, but is now healthy and doing very well, I'm happy to say.

She'd opted for a bilateral mastectomy with tissue expanders. She hadn't had radiation, so there wasn't that added complication that I had to deal with.

We talked about my recurrence, and she laid this little bombshell on me: "Margaret, I'm just putting this out there, but what if you get the single mastectomy and it comes back on the other side? Then you'd have to go through it all over again."

My world, and my head, began to spin.

She continued, "My friend Patty had breast cancer; she went through a mastectomy on one side, chemotherapy, then it came back on the other side two years later. She was absolutely devastated."

For sure.

"But my other side is fine," I told her. "And they'll watch it closely. I see my oncologist every six months anyway. She keeps an eye on me."

Sally paused to regroup before continuing.

"I'll tell you what my doctor said to me: 'Taking the other breast is like amputating a healthy arm. Why would you do that?' But I had him take both anyway, and when they got the pathology report back, he told me there were abnormal cells on the good side."

Crap.

Things got real again. My world felt like it had gone completely topsy-turvy.

One was bad enough, but two?

I called my oncologist, Dr. Rossi, to get her opinion, leaving a message with her nurse. While I waited for her to return my call, I thought to myself: I was thirty-four with my first diagnosis, forty-six with the second. Did I really want to go through this again at fifty-eighty?

And then there was the cyst and biopsy procedure I'd been through two years before with Righty, my good breast, which had come back negative but had given me a week's worth of worry.

If I didn't have both breasts removed, would I always have the thought of breast cancer lingering at the back of my mind?

Dr. Rossi returned my call, giving me the pros and cons. Her argument against the bilateral: "We'll keep a close eye on you. You'll have your annual mammograms on that side, and we'll catch it early if anything's going on."

Her pros for removing both: "No follow-up treatment, no chemotherapy, no radiation, no pills." And the plastic surgeon would be better able to create uniformity.

Also, I'd been given the option of genetic testing to see whether my BRCA1 or BRCA2 genes showed mutations indicating a higher risk of breast cancer, which could be an indication for choosing a preventive mastectomy.

I weighed the pros and cons.

Ultimately, it was a roll of the dice. I could go the rest of my life with Righty and be just fine. Or not. I wouldn't know for sure if Righty had any signs of cancer until after she was gone. There were no guarantees.

I thought about losing both my breasts, Lefty, the Troublemaker, and Righty, the Good One.

I decided to have both breasts removed.

So You Find Out You're Losing Both Of Your Breasts

As soon as you trust yourself, you will know how to live.
~ *J.W. von Goethe*

I was strangely calm. Maybe because I'd been living all these years knowing that there was a possibility of recurrence, so it wasn't a complete and utter shock like it was the first time. My good friend Bob had once shared with me, years ago, that his mother was a breast cancer survivor, twice. She had it on one side, had a mastectomy, then went through it again years later on the other side.

It's funny how one comment can remain in the recesses of one's brain.

Bob's mother is still with us, thankfully, and thriving these many years later. But you live your life, you go on, and after twelve years, truthfully, it wasn't on my radar. More temporal matters were my focus—where my next paying job would come from, day-to-day hassles like paying the bills or running errands for my mother-in-law who'd stopped driving.

2012 was the year I'd have my first book published, and as anyone who's put their heart and soul into a project knows, it can become all-encompassing. So there was work; my book; there was Andrew, whose high school schedule was so busy that keeping up with it was like a full-time job, with Steve and I playing support roles. The bilateral mastectomy wasn't something I had time for. Almost immediately, though, once I'd gotten my mind worked out that I'd do it, it became the forefront of my life, looming large. Very large.

I had long conversations with my oldest sister, Mary, a veterinarian with a scientific brain and vast medical knowledge. She grilled me over the whys, demanding, in her alpha oldest sister way, to know why remove two breasts when I could simply take one?

It was a valid question.

Preventive. That's all I could say.

There isn't necessarily a right answer, unless your cancer type has a very strong risk of appearing on the other side.

Mary couldn't talk me out of it. My mind was made up. Sort of.

———

Climbing Mountains (Or Very Large Hills)

Go big or go home. Because it's true. What do you have to lose?

~ Eliza Dushku

With the surgery date only a month away, my sister Mary had a plan: she'd come down for a weekend of fun—and when a person is facing something as crappy as a bilateral mastectomy, fun is desperately needed—and for my birthday would take me, my sisters, and our mom to see Bruce Springsteen at the Sports Arena.

My sister Mary is dynamic, to say the least, and has been known to sometimes bully her way around. Just a bit. I've learned not to say no to her. (And why would I say no to The Boss anyway?)

It was a great night.

The next day, because Mary didn't want to sit around and talk about my cancer, she, our sister Kathy, my niece April, Andrew, and I made a trip to Griffith Park in which alpha Mary decided we would hike up the mountain.

Hike up.

Up.

A mountain. (Or hill in the case of Griffith Park.)

I'm not a mountain climber, let me just get that out there, but here I was, having just celebrated my forty-seventh birthday, looking ahead to my bilateral mastec-tomy with a large amount of apprehension; single-mindedly focused on getting it over with. I knew the sur-gery would be significant, performed by two teams of sur-geons: first, my general surgeon, Dr. Mandelbaum, who would do the actual breast removal; followed by my plas-tic surgeon, Dr. Hill, and her team, who would put the tissue expanders in place.

The estimated length of surgery was four to five hours. Surprisingly, my stay in the hospital would only be overnight unless complications arose.

But back to the climbing part.

Now, I guess I can *sort of* get why people climb Mt. Everest or any other high place. They eventually slog their way up through the challenging topography and thin air to the very top so they can then look out and appreciate the view and all they've accomplished.

But me? I'm a flatlander. I don't mind walking or hiking *necessarily*, as long as it's flattish. It's my slacker makeup, my desire to take the path of least resistance. This is me. This is who I am. And another thing: L.A. can be very hot in the springtime. Hiking plus heat equals an unhappy me. But then there was the matter of my sister Mary and her will of iron.

So we walked up one of the many dirt trails at Griffith Park, passing lots of people wearing varying degrees of clothing—workout clothes, short-shorts, tank tops—carrying bottled water, walking all varieties of dogs. The sun beat down. A hot flash kicked in. I sweated. Then another hot flash. My loyal niece April stayed behind with me, dutifully and cheerfully, as I complained.

My sisters laughed at me.

Andrew laughed at me.

"You guys *suck!*" I railed up the trail towards them.

They still laughed, looking down on me from their vantage point above us, mocking me with their superior hiking skills.

Eventually, we made it to the top. And the view from the Griffith Park Observatory is one of the best in Los Angeles. The sky was bright blue, the clouds were puffy and white. We wandered around the great expanse of lawn in front of the observatory, looked at the Astronomers Monument featuring Copernicus, Galileo, Newton, and the other scientific greats. We browsed the exhibits inside, and took in a planetarium show, which is always a good reminder of our status as humans in the scheme of things.

We are little specks, passing through. We are stardust.

I'd climbed the mountain (or hill), and it was totally worth it.

Genetic Counseling

Science never solves a problem without creating ten more.

~ George Bernard Shaw

By the time my appointment with the genetic counselor had been made, I'd already decided to have both breasts removed. The testing was more for my sisters and nieces, to let them know about any risk they might have so they could get themselves checked out if my test came back positive.

The more I learned about the genetic testing, the more I realized it's another numbers game. And it's very complex. When I'd mentioned it to my friend Sally, she confided that she'd been tested too, and that her test had come back negative; yet, her other breast still showed signs of cancer when it was removed.

When I met with my genetic counselor, she explained, going into great detail, the testing process. Basically, what I learned was that the test was an indicator only—a very specific indicator—and not a guarantee one way or the other. (Insert heavy sigh here.)

Without getting too complex—because my head will start to hurt soon if I do—I was sent to the lab at Kaiser where a blood sample was taken. The sample was then sent to a lab in Utah to be analyzed. Three weeks later, the lab sent their findings back to my genetic counselor at Kaiser. My results were negative. Good news for my sisters and nieces, but I remained unchanged in my decision to have both breasts removed.

[To learn more about BRCA1 and BRCA2 testing, visit the National Cancer Institute: http://www.cancer.gov/cancertopics/factsheet/Risk/BRCA

To learn about the related BART test, visit Breastcancer.org, dedicated to providing reliable, complete, and up-to-date information about breast cancer: http://www.breastcancer.org/symptoms/testing/genetic/facility_cost]

Goodbye To My Old Friends

If you live to be a hundred, I want to be a hundred minus one day so I never have to live without you.
~ *A.A. Milne*

Steve and I left the house early, about five a.m., on the day of my surgery. Andrew would be on his own and had set his alarm to get himself to school.

I waited in line at the surgery check-in, playing a little game: try to spot the surgery patient versus their loved one/companion. It wasn't too hard to tell the patients; we were the ones wearing no jewelry, not carrying purses, the ones wearing slippers, the ones that looked slightly apprehensive. Pretty easy tells.

The woman at the desk took my Kaiser card and told me it would cost $500—my hospital copay. Thank God we'd managed to hang on to our health insurance. (Don't get me started on affordable health care.)

Steve called Andrew at six-thirty to make sure he was up for school, and I waited for the nurse to take me back to pre-op.

Once I changed into my pre-op gown, they put those little boot thingies on my feet and calves to keep the circulation going during surgery so blood clots wouldn't form. My gown was extra quilty, not a typical hospital gown. It even had a little tube attached to a heater so I could stay warm.

The nurse who cared for me before surgery was named Leyna. Originally from Singapore, she was older, calm and reassuring, with a lovely low voice. She was friendly, and we laughed about things—what, I have no idea. She was just the kind of person you'd want attending to you before undergoing such a sucky thing.

After I answered all of Leyna's questions—the long list of "Do you have this? Do you have that?" to best ensure that I'd actually make it through the procedure just fine—yes, please!—Leyna brought Steve back so he could sit with me until they rolled me away.

The first thing I noticed when he walked up was his reassuring smile. My steady partner sat next to my bed, just as he had twelve years before, and held my hand.

He'd been tested over the years.

When I was twenty-three weeks pregnant with Andrew and had early contractions, the doctors thought I'd deliver my baby at one and a half pounds. I spent three days in ICU on a magnesium sulfate drip to stop the contractions. Steve stood by me then, making calls, grabbing anyone who passed by, cross-examining doctors—making sure I was being taken care of properly.

He stood by me through the five months of pregnancy bed rest, taking care of me, the house, grocery shopping—everything. Then later, he stood by me every step of the way with my first breast cancer diagnosis.

Now this. This was a man who took his marriage vows seriously. There's not much more I can say than that, is there?

He sat with me in the pre-op area, holding my hand, joking about the little things that we'd laugh at as a couple. I'd make him laugh too, because humor is what you really need; it's the thing that can help you in a situation like this. Really.

Dr. Mandelbaum, my general surgeon, stopped by to give me his thumbs up. I liked him—a big bear of a man, with a kind bedside manner. When we'd met for my pre-op appointment and I told him about my decision to have both breasts removed, he nodded, saying, "I think you're doing the right thing." I have a feeling he would have said the same thing if I told him I was planning to have a single mastectomy, but still, his support helped.

Next, the anesthesiologist stopped by to introduce himself. I told him I'd had trouble with anesthesia before, hoping he could do anything so I wouldn't vomit after surgery. He said something like, "I'll put something in your IV."

Dr. Hill, the petite plastic surgeon who reminded me of the actress Lisa Hartman Black, stopped by to say hello before she changed into her scrubs. She was wearing what looked to be workout clothes, her hair was damp. She was pumped and ready to go.

I took a deep breath and squeezed Steve's hand. The nurse gave me something to relax, and then I didn't care about anything anymore. Steve squeezed my hand this time, and they wheeled me away to the O.R.

Wait, What?

**That which does
not kill us makes
us stronger.**
~ *Friedrich Nietzsche*

When I woke up in post-op, I don't remember feeling
pain. Leyna, my kind pre-op nurse, checked me over,
instructing me how to give myself more morphine—which is a dangerous thing. All I had to do was
clickety-click the handy little button, and I planned to,
just like a monkey. My thumb was ready.

I hadn't had any nausea and was lying there trying to
focus. Soon Steve was sitting by my side. He'd spoken to
the surgeons; everything had gone well.

I didn't look down towards my chest; I didn't care at
this point, being heavily medicated.

Steve and I laughed; we chatted. I don't have much memory about any of this until a young nurse arrived to wheel my bed to my hospital room.

Away we went, rolling down the hall, around the corner, into a room with its own hospital bed.

Wait. What?

I remember thinking: *Huh. How is the bed I'm lying on going to fit in the room? There's not enough space for two beds.*

"Okay," the energetic young nurse said, "we're going to have to transfer you."

Oh, no. You didn't just say that, did you?

It was funny, but it sounded like she'd said I'd have to move. My body. Over there.

It was like one of those cartoon moments where the character's eyes pop right out of their head, making that little "awoo-ga" sound.

You are totally shitting me; right?

Me: "You mean I'm going to have to *move?*"

Her: "Yes."

Me: "To that bed *there?*"

Her: "Yes. We'll do it in stages."

Getting my mind wrapped around this little bomb-shell was kind of like when I was in labor with my son and the nurse informed me that I wouldn't be getting my epidural; that I was way past that.

The transfer happened, I somehow made it onto the hospital bed, and it felt like someone was sawing my back. Literally, it felt as if a tiny man was slowly sawing the back of my shoulder with a hand saw. Burning pain. The opposite of good. I don't know why I was having pain in my back and not my front; I just was.

Luckily the extreme pain only lasted a few seconds. (Let us not forget the morphine and my little hand on the button.)

The thing about morphine, though, is that while it relieves pain, it can make a person sick. So while I wasn't in much pain while I was on it, I couldn't keep anything down.

Dr. Hill had mentioned that I probably wouldn't feel like eating much the first day or two after surgery, and they didn't bring me any real food the first day, but I had juice and Jell-O. I'd sip the juice, and twenty minutes later, I'd bring it back up.

Retching, after having had the surgery I'd had, is pretty much the opposite of what we humans like to think of as a good time. Yet, I threw up all day, and late into the night. Anything that went down came back up again.

Finally, after I'd complained to every nurse who would listen, I was taken off the morphine and switched to a pill pain reliever, Norco. The vomiting went away, thank the Lord.

This was not an easy time for me, with the first twelve hours in my hospital bed post-surgery being the roughest. So this is where I give special thanks to my dear sister Kathy for staying with me overnight.

I didn't think I'd need babysitting and urged Steve to go home to be with Andrew. My sweet sister Jenny, who'd brought a plate of cookies, which I gave to the nursing staff so they'd hopefully treat me better—and, no, I am not above bribery—went home in the late afternoon, along with my friend Pamela, who'd also stayed all day.

It is a *very* good thing to have someone stay with you after you've had surgery, especially if you're not mobile yet. I wasn't able to get out of bed—the thought of it was pretty much beyond comprehension—and the constant IV drip of normal saline into my veins made me have to "go" frequently, which meant using a bed pan.

It was hard enough managing to fit the pan under me when every little movement had the potential for extreme discomfort. I'd have to grab a nurse each time, first to request the bedpan and then to empty it. (I think I needed to do this just about every forty-five minutes to an hour.) Most of the nurses were good-natured about this, but once when I asked the first nurse I saw—one I hadn't seen before—she gave me a death stare, and I felt small. I mean, I felt like I was five years old and the neighbor lady was chewing me out because I'd blown up the inflatable giraffe sitting on her coffee table without her permission.

But I *really* had to go.

What was I supposed to do? Wet myself and the bed?

After feeling ashamed and humiliated, having to humble myself before this witch for my bed pan, feeling crappy about having to keep finding nurses the rest of the night, sister Kathy appeared out of nowhere. She'd gone home to take care of her bunnies—she owns a herd of the fuzzy little creatures—and after she returned, she emptied my bed pan all night, even waking up to do it when I whisper-called her name so I wouldn't startle her.

If that isn't love, I don't know what is.

They gave me a sleeping pill that night, but my body seemed to have just shaken it off. Sleep eluded me, so during the long night in the hospital, I kept telling myself: *This is only temporary. Every hour that passes, I'll be that much less sore.*

It was a very long night, but then it was over.

Time passes; time heals.

Before I knew it, Steve was there taking a picture of me—I could do nothing to stop him—as I grimaced and held onto half of the turkey sandwich I'd been brought for lunch. For the longest time, I couldn't bear to look at this picture where I'm puffy and look completely miserable, my "souvenir" of the whole ghastly experience. I was ready to go home.

Needless to say, the car ride home was rough; every bump hurt, but the pillows Steve brought, which we propped around, under, and about me, helped.

Handy hospital check list:

1. Have someone bring treats for the nurses so they'll hopefully be a little nicer to you. This can be as simple as a bag of Hershey's kisses or peanut butter cups.

You can also have someone place a bowl of treats on your bedside table to offer to anyone who comes into your room. Bribery in the form of treats is perfectly legal and acceptable.

2. Try to arrange for a relative or close friend to spend the night in the hospital with you in case you need help with your bedpans and other little niceties, since you probably won't be ambulatory at first.

3. Bring an oversized shirt that buttons in the front for the ride home. This is important. You will *not* want to have to slip anything over your head. Trust me. I chose a Hawaiian shirt from the thrift store, one I'd picked up during a special trip just for shirts that buttoned in the front. (This probably explains my current anti-Hawaiian shirt bias.) You'll want extra shirts that button in the front. Men's shirts also work well.

4. Have your driver bring pillows for comfort on the ride home so you'll feel fewer of the bumps along the way.

5. Before surgery, give yourself a pedicure because you won't be able to do that for quite a while afterwards. At least your toes will look good.

The first few days at home post-surgery saw me mostly camped out on the bed. Steve had created this ingenious little support mountain using pillows, a rolled-up comforter, and blankets, wedged against the headboard, so I'd be able to sit and sleep in a propped-up position.

Some women who undergo mastectomies will sleep in a recliner for several weeks. I looked into this option and couldn't get my mind around paying $250 to $300 to rent one for a month. (I'd been out of work for a few weeks and saw unemployment in my immediate future.)

I'd been given pain medication, Tylenol 3 with codeine, which made me sleepy, so lying on my bed and pillow mountain, for the first few days at least, sleep wasn't too difficult.

I took my pain medication every four hours, ate yogurt*, Jell-O, and sipped broth.

My second day post-op, I felt much better. I was still confined to bed, and Andrew hung out with me. This fact alone is remarkable: my fourteen-year-old teenager stayed with his *mother* all day. It was the Sunday of Memorial Day weekend, and A&E was airing a marathon of the show "Oddities," of all things. So we watched the "Oddities" marathon, or I watched and Andrew played Angry Birds on his phone.

This was the same boy who tried to be born much too early; the same boy who'd grown up with my oncology appointments, carefully questioning me about each one, looking for reassurance; the same boy I'd had so many heart-to-heart conversations with God about.

Andrew stayed by my side, and by his simple presence, not saying much, just being there, we gave each other the silent assurance that everything would be okay.

[**Tip:** *Yogurt probably wasn't the best idea because the anesthesia in combination with the morphine made me extremely constipated, and sometimes milk products can exacerbate an already slow digestive system. Of course, I wouldn't know this for a few days. I should have been eating things with more of a laxative effect. Having prune juice handy wouldn't be a bad idea in this circumstance. Also ginger ale in case of stomach upset. Ginger ale containing real ginger is even better. Check the label.]*

Let Me Get This Off My Chest

A Word About Drains, And Bras With Special Attachments

The best things in life are unexpected—because there were no expectations.

~ *Eli Khamarov*

About two weeks before my mastectomy surgery, I was given a referral from Kaiser to a special boutique—one that dealt specifically with women with breast cancer and their issues. My insurance would cover the cost of two bras.

Dr. Hill had instructed me to show up on the day of surgery with a front-closing sports bra.

I made my appointment with the bra store and once there soon found myself naked from the waist up in a fitting room with my very own salesclerk/bra consultant who measured me for the exact right bra. I sat there as she held the tape up to my chest, and I listened to her talk about her own breast cancer scare, nodding the whole time, but really just wanting to get my bras and go. It was very warm inside the store, and I had a hot flash, and I soon broke out into an all-over-the-body sweat.

The cool thing about my experience was that the special bra had these little bags that attached with Velcro to the front of the bra where I could put my drains post-surgery, allowing me to move freely and not worry about having to carry them, with the tubing getting in the way.

They say it's the little things, but, really, this was a big load off, a wonderful invention, and something every woman who undergoes a mastectomy should have. The bras were expensive, $108 for two of them, but, as I said, insurance covered it. They would have been worth the

price even if I would have had to pay the full amount
myself.

Dr. Hill instructed me that post-surgery, the sports
bra and I, we'd be very close friends—very close—with
me wearing it 24/seven, only taking it off to shower and
put the antibiotic cream on my incisions.

My surgery had left me with one drain on each side. Basically, the drain is a long tube with a bulb at the end
where the lymph and excess fluid ends up. I was instructed to empty the drains into a little cup and keep
track of the output. Once I hit a certain number and the
output had slowed—I think it was ten milliliters in a
twenty-four-hour period—the drains could come out.

This really wasn't as bad as it sounds; a minor pain,
but not *too* bad. I had a small opening on each side of the
chest, towards my back—about two inches down from
where my breasts used to be—where the tubes came out.
The openings were just large enough for the tubes to fit
through.

My surgery happened on a Friday, I was out of the
hospital Saturday, and by the following Thursday—so
after six days—my drains were removed.

The drain removal happened at my second post-op appointment. (My first appointment on the Monday following surgery is hazy. It hurt to walk, I know I was wincing in pain with every step, and I'm sure the people sitting in the waiting area looked upon me with much pity.)

Having the drains taken out was something to celebrate. It didn't hurt at all—just a small tug on each side as I held my breath for a second and Dr. Hill pulled—and we did celebrate by stopping at the little tamale place on the way home from Kaiser.

I waited in the car as Steve ran inside and bought a dozen tamales. Things were starting to look up, even if they weren't tacos*.

[*I have a special relationship with tacos.]

Medications May Need To Be Adjusted

Sometimes I say the medication is even tougher than the illness.

~ *Sanya Richards-Ross*

One week post-surgery, I saw Dr. Mandelbaum, the general surgeon. Before my surgery, I'd requested Tylenol 3 with codeine for the pain. The codeine did make me sleepy, which was good, but it didn't do as much for the pain as I thought it would, so Dr. Mandelbaum wrote me scrip for Norco, an opiate derivative. The generic form is hydrocodone.

Dr. Mandelbaum was happy to see me, happy with how I was doing. He took a look at my in-progress breasts, peering under the remaining mountain of gauze and bandages, and I asked him, more out of curiosity than anything else, if the pathology report had shown any cancer on the right side—the good, non-cancer side. He shook his head, simply saying no, and moving on.

I felt my stomach turn. My feelings at this point are a little hard to explain. I felt conflicting emotions: happy that there wasn't more cancer because no cancer is always better. Always. But then there was the other side of my thoughts: *So I didn't need to have the right breast taken.*

But why bother second-guessing yourself when the deed has been done? Why in the world would I bother beating myself up about it?

Dr. Mandelbaum must have sensed my internal conflict, imagining the tortured machinations going on in that hamster wheel in my brain, because he looked at me, with a look of kindness and compassion that I will never forget, and said, "You made the right decision."

Thank you, Dr. Mandelbaum. I have big fuzzy hugs for you.

Now, a few more words about Norco. (See also: constipation.)

Hydrocodone is known to be habit-forming and, in my opinion, it seems to be prescribed a little bit too often. So if you find yourself with a prescription, be careful. Proceed with caution.

I took one Norco tablet, and I was whacked. It made me feel all loopy, woozy, lightheaded, and very, very sleepy. I didn't like it at all, so I put the bottle away and went back to my Tylenol with codeine.

When my friend Sally called to check in, I complained about the Norco and its effects on me.

"Cut it in half," she said simply.

Duh!

I felt like an idiot when she told me this. Makes sense; right?

So Steve went out and bought a pill splitter—a very good one—from the Walgreens around the corner from us, and I started cutting the Norco in half. I still didn't use too many—maybe one or two halves a day—but found that it was enough to manage the pain.

I soon discovered, though, if I took the Norco too many days in a row, it wreaked havoc on my digestive system. So, again, use with caution.

Now, getting back to the, ahem, constipation. The combination of anesthesia, morphine, and probably the codeine from the Tylenol 3, slowed my digestion to a crawl. Less than a crawl. Nothing was moving. (You know what I mean, people. Don't make me have to say it.)

So on Tuesday night, five days post-op, it probably wasn't the *best* idea to have a big, home-cooked meal, but Steve, being the wonderful, caring husband that he is, decided to give me a real feast. He barbecued, made some lovely fresh spinach, a salad, fruit, mashed potatoes, and a crusty sourdough roll. I ate my dinner in bed, watching an episode of the miniseries "Hatfields & McCoys." Everything was delicious, but about twenty minutes after eating, I started to feel nausea accompanied by sharp knife pains in my gut—the kind that usually signal that a trip to the bathroom is imminent. I started sipping ginger ale to quell the nauseous feelings. It would help for a minute or two, the nausea would subside, and then the knife pains would start again.

I'd hobble off to the bathroom, and nothing. The pains and nausea went on for hours, making for one terrible, awful, horrible night. Nothing budged. It felt like the food was rotting in my stomach, not passing through to the intestines, and I was horribly full and uncomfortable.

Steve ran out to the drugstore the next morning and brought back Mylanta*. I immediately took a dose, and then another dose a few hours later.

I did this for three long days, and then I—well, you know.

Word to the wise: don't have a big meal after a major surgery until things are, um, moving again.

Trust me on this one.

This handy bit of advice may also be filed under the heading of: Things doctors don't tell you. (But they really should.)

[*Tip:* *Having Mylanta in the house would probably be a good idea post-surgery. Also, prune juice and other fruit juices, bran cereal, even a fiber supplement like Metamucil in case your digestive system needs a little nudge.*]

The Deep Dark Places, The Lonely Nights

We have to go into the despair and go beyond it, by working and doing for somebody else, by using it for something else.

~ *Elie Wiesel*

In the days and weeks following surgery, my body healed slowly. I took things very easy the first few days, burning through the different cable stations, watching cooking shows, home design shows, talk shows, looking for movies. I learned quickly: there is nothing worth watching on television during the day. Fifty-million cable channels; nothing on. So I read a lot of books, wrote on my laptop in spurts—overdoing it—talked on the phone, and spent a lot of time either on my bed or on the couch.

Tissue expanders are not comfortable. Since they're temporary implants designed to be expanded gradually, they're thicker than regular implants and give the skin a ripply feel. My chest muscles and in-progress breasts were now higher up on my chest, and my good side, where Righty was, had pain under the arm which radiated around to my back and the side of my shoulder. Ironically, my left side was fine. The preponderance of my pain was situated on my non-cancer prophylactic mastectomy side. (But I will *try* not to sound bitter.)

Throughout this time Steve did everything—housework, laundry, shopping, cooking. I quickly learned not to fuss about the little things. I ignored the constant tufts of white fur that our Australian Shepherd, Chance, casts off daily, or Andrew's full laundry hamper and the clothes spilling onto the floor.

Letting go of things like housework can be difficult; I've, uh, heard other women have this problem too. We want to control things; we want them to be done the way *we* want them done. And it's stupid, really. Not sweating the little things helped to minimize stress, not only on myself, but on Steve who was trying to do his best. So maybe he didn't fold the laundry like I did, or maybe he scrambled eggs differently. Life did go on; the Earth continued to spin. The up side was that I was able to heal, and someone was helping to facilitate that process.

At first, sleeping propped up on my back wasn't *too* bad—I was fairly drugged-up the first two weeks—but by week five, the stress on my back from remaining in a fixed position at night was starting to take its toll.

Once given the clear by Dr. Hill, at about six weeks post-surgery, I began tentatively trying to sleep on my side. Very gently, rolling ever-so-slightly on one side or the other. This helped, believe it or not, to relieve the pressure on my lower back.

Nights were hard, though. Trying to get comfortable was challenging in and of itself. I'd also have hot flashes, first throwing my comforter off, then my blanket, then top sheet.

Not having a work schedule, and not getting up to take Andrew to school in the morning gave me this feeling of amorphousness, of floating through life without any other purpose than passing the time, waiting as my body healed. I found myself staying up later and later, staring up at the ceiling, not falling asleep until three or four in the morning. In those sleepless hours, my wide-awake mind traveled to the really dark places.

There were the dark places of self-doubt where I'd roll over in my mind every failure, cataloguing them, counting the ways in which I'd disappointed myself. Then there were the dark places of worry and fear about my future, about whether I'd be able to return to work as a court reporter. I worried about my bills, which seemed to be having babies, reproducing at an alarming rate, and there was nothing I could do to stop them. There is no such thing as bill birth control.

My personal challenge was, and is, to not let those fears take over and let them take residence in my head.

Worry, worry, worry.

And one other important thing about cancer or any other serious illness, it's your own "thing." No one can endure the pain and discomfort for you, as much as they'd like to. My mother, mother-in-law, Steve, my sisters—they all wished to take my place, which is pretty selfless of them. Still, it was my own journey, which is a little bit of a sobering thought. It felt isolating sometimes, the different mental and physical issues I was working with, working through.

It's a normal thing, going through something like cancer, to have depressing thoughts. When my mind would go to those very dark places, I would try to redirect and think of something good—my son, my husband, my mom, my sisters, my friends. Thankfully, I don't have to think too hard to come up with a good thing. There is always *something* to be happy about. It comes back to the matter of perspective and the realization that things could be worse. (They could.)

I wish I had a perfect, tidy answer to help others when they feel like their mind is dwelling too much in those dark places, but all I have are suggestions.

Call a friend, call your mom, call your dad. If it's the middle of the night, like so many of my trips to the dark places have been, then get your journal out and write. Or type an e-mail to a friend, save it as a draft, and send it the next day.

If it feels like the depression, fears, and anxiety are getting the best of you, though, tell your doctor.

Losing one's breast(s) is a big deal emotionally and physically. The dark places are normal; you just don't want to let them take over.

[CancerCare.org provides free support and counseling services for people dealing with all types of cancers: http://www.cancercare.org/counseling]

Frankenboobs

**There is a kind
of beauty in
imperfection.**
~ *Conrad Hall*

Hopped-up on pain killers immediately following my
double mastectomy and reconstruction, I didn't care
what was under my hospital gown, which seems a little
funny in retrospect. My breasts were gone, but I was too
numb to be in mourning. What I somehow managed to
comprehend below my hospital gown, below my special
fancy sports bra with the front hooks and little drain
compartments, was large amounts of gauze. It looked as
if my stuffing was coming out.

Upon discharge from the hospital, I was instructed
not to shower—sponge baths only—until given the all
clear. Now, the no-shower edict was not a problem see-

ing as how I was in move-as-little-as-possible mode. A shower wasn't a priority; staying in one place and concentrating on not being in pain or discomfort was at the top of my list.

During my first Monday appointment post-surgery, Dr. Hill removed some of the gauze, leaving just enough to cover the steri strips over my incisions, which were long, four-inch uneven lines cutting across the middle of each breast. When Dr. Hill removed the extra gauze, I didn't even look down; somehow, I wasn't ready to see what things looked like there.

At my visit three days later, Dr. Hill removed the rest of the dressing, giving me little gauze squares to put inside my bra to cover and protect my incisions.

Now, something I'd kept in mind up to this point was a comment my friend Sally made when describing her post double mastectomy tissue expander chest.

"That's some trippy shit going on there," she'd warned me.

She was totally right. The "trippy shit" to which she was referring was the work-in-progress look of the whole freaky thing. When I was looking ahead to my upcoming mastectomy, the way Sally had described feeling detached from her reconstruction gave me comfort. Being a modest person, she would never have dreamt of lifting her shirt to show someone her breasts, but it was different with her reconstructed ones, as if they were some abstract lab experiment or something. During her reconstruction process, she found herself lifting her shirt to show her new breasts to people with little or no prompting.

What I found after the gauze had been taken away (leaving just the clear steri strips): my incisions were angry-looking and dark with dried blood. I had purple and yellow bruises over the tops and undersides of my new breasts, as well as stray bruises on my back and shoulders. Lefty, the Troublemaker, was now higher up on my chest than Righty, my noncancerous breast. My right breast had a strange look, as if there was too much skin left over. It was kind of puckered, or twisted, under itself. During surgery, the left side had been filled with 100 cc's of saline; the right side had 150 cc's. They were lopsided.

I had very small beginning breasts. I had Frankenboobs. Not pretty, but they were a start.

Let Me Get This Off My Chest

Dr. Hill's plan was to fill my tissue expanders every two to three weeks, slowly adding saline to Lefty to prevent complications.

Slowly, slowly, we'd proceed, my Frankenboobs and me.

Saline Fills

I dwell in possibility.
~ *Emily Dickinson*

My first saline fill was a month post-surgery. I'd been advised to take a couple of Tylenols beforehand. I'd also spent time scaring myself—I mean researching—reading about other women's experiences with saline fills. The consensus on the breast cancer forums was that the fills are one of those things where it really depends on the individual. Some women found them very uncomfortable, while others found them to be no big deal. Some women complained about getting too much saline injected at one time and having to have some drawn off because their breasts felt too stretched and uncomfortable, while others sailed through the process.

Naturally, after spending time reading the different accounts, I felt a little apprehensive. And my experience calls to mind the conventional wisdom that goes something like: never research important medical things on the Internet because you will soon convince yourself that you will die. Scraped knee? Death. Hurt elbow? Certain death.

In actuality—real life—what I found was that the first twenty-four hours after my first saline fill were the most uncomfortable, but that the Tylenol taken beforehand probably helped because I didn't have too much discomfort immediately afterward. Dr. Hill took a conservative approach, filling 60 cc's on the radiated side and 75 cc's on the non-radiated right side.

Each visit, a nurse would take me into a room which was basically a very large exam room with a long table in the center and overhead lights. The nurse—usually a very nice older woman, Sharon—would have me lie down on the table, with a pillow underneath my head, and prep the area of my chest, washing it with antiseptic wipes. Dr. Hill would then come in and chat with me as she'd first give me a numbing shot, then locate the little port in the implant using a small magnet. Next, using a fat syringe, she would slowly inject the fluid. This process didn't hurt, but I did have a sensation of fullness as the saline entered the tissue expanders.

This fill procedure was repeated every few weeks for a total of five fills, and the subsequent fills became much more comfortable as I went along. At the end of the process, I had 350 and 375 milliliters of fluid in each tissue expander.

Now, a loose rule of thumb when figuring out cup size is: 200 cc's of fluid equals one cup size. So my 375 cc's equaled fairly solid B cups.

My former breast cup had been C, but the size wasn't important to me. At every stage of the expansion process, I reminded Dr. Hill I would be happy with small breasts. I wasn't looking at getting a free breast augmentation out of the deal; I didn't need large breasts. I just wanted something to fill my bra and help me to feel a little bit like my old self.

The radiated breast all along, though, seemed to have a mind of its own. Lefty, in other words, continued to be a troublemaker, and with each fill, the fluid would kind of go where it wanted to go, leaving me with a temporary breast that was large on the top but with hardly anything underneath except for a strange indentation where the fluid *didn't* go. The effect was not one of uniformity; it was just strange-looking.

My Frankenboobs were looking more Frankenboobish all the time.

[**Tip:** *Take a pain reliever approved by your doctor—an over-the-counter is probably all you'll need—before you have your saline fills. This will help alleviate any post-saline fill discomfort.*]

Catching My Breath

Smile, breathe, and go slowly.
~ *Thich Nhat Hanh*

One thing I wasn't prepared for, that kind of caught me off guard, was my lack of breath following my bilateral mastectomy. It wasn't a shortness of breath so much as a feeling that I couldn't draw a deep breath; my breathing had become shallow.

Dr. Hill had warned me that after surgery, there wouldn't be pain so much as a feeling of fullness or tightness. (Someone else compared it to the feeling of having an elephant sitting in the middle of one's chest, but I wouldn't go that far.)

While I was in the hospital, I was given a breathing device and advised to use it once an hour, sucking on the little tube attachment that would bring up the float inside, working the lungs. (It is very important.)

Having the breathing tube inserted during the surgery, combined with being under anesthesia for an extended period of time, along with the tightness across my chest from the operation itself, inhibited my ability to take a deep breath, which led to my feeling of being easily winded in the days and weeks following surgery.

As I gradually improved, day by day, in little increments, using my breathing treatment, I did feel myself getting my hot air back. (If you were to talk to Steve, he'd probably say it never left, and then he'd laugh an evil laugh because that's the way he is.)

One thing I noticed, though, was that when I started to walk, my lung function seemed to improve much more quickly. On the 4th of July—so about five and a half weeks post-surgery—I was very brave and decided to walk up to the end of the street with Andrew, up to the school on the corner, to check out the annual 4th of July carnival. This was my biggest walk to date and probably amounted to a total of a half mile, up and back. The carnival itself was nothing more than those rickety traveling rides, corn dogs, scary-looking carnies, and kettle corn—not too exciting—but it did let me know that I could do it. I could walk actual distances, *and* I could get my own kettle corn.

When we returned home, I rested from my big excursion, and the next day I laced up my running shoes—which I knew wouldn't be used for running any time in my foreseeable future—and walked up to the school, first intending to walk half the length around it but then pushing myself to do the whole thing. This walk was just over a mile. I did that for the next few days and felt like I'd turned a corner; my breathing was becoming easier.

In the midst of this, I started daily yoga stretches after Dr. Hill gave me permission, walked a little more, and felt like I was returning to my old self, if just a little.

[**Tip:** *The little breathing apparatus I was given in the hospital I later learned is called a* **spirometer**. *If you're given one of these devices, you'll most likely take it home from the hospital with you. Use it for a few days once you're home; it will help to improve your breathing function. Don't forget to use it while in the hospital. This is important, and your nurses may not remind you. I was on my own with this, and I'm glad I used it.*]

Let Me Get This Off My Chest

[*sex]

I don't know the question, but sex is definitely the answer.

~ *Woody Allen*

First, give yourself ten points if you flipped ahead to this chapter before reading anything else. (Naughty!)

Now, take ten points away if you were expecting something raunchy. (This isn't *50 Shades of Grey*, people. Not much.)

Back in 1999 and the beginning of 2000 when Steve and I were getting our honorary Ph.D.'s in cancer research online and were doing all we could to learn about what it was he and I would be going through together, we learned something surprising: apparently the rate of divorce is fairly high among couples where one of the spouses has been diagnosed with cancer.

This thought made my brain hurt. What about the vows? The sickness and health part? How could this be? The very idea seemed so sad and cruel to me, and Steve and I very seriously told each other this wouldn't happen to us. Not *us*.

But cancer can be a wedge in a relationship. Some people simply aren't good dealing with medical issues; maybe they're not naturally empathetic, or maybe they don't know how to react when the spouse with cancer is having a crying jag and her emotions are a jumbly, mascara-smearing mess.

This is real.

Even the best of us, with our angel wings and halos, can be trying to be around. I know, this is hard to imagine, but even I felt my usually calm self turn into a psycho nut when I was having a moment. Even I have felt like I needed to apologize at times to my dear partner because I'd gotten a little emotionally out of control.

It's important to stay physically and emotionally connected to your partner, to keep the intimacy going because the longer you go without having sex, the easier it is to let things slide and not have it. Pretty soon, you're in the midst of a sexual desert, lost and adrift. Frustrated. Thirsty. Sad.

Sex was definitely *not* on my radar in the first few weeks post-mastectomy. Not only was I in way too much discomfort, I had the whole issue of my tissue expanders, and stitches. Let's not forget my Frankenboobs.

Somewhere around week five or six, when I started walking distances again and was feeling a bit more like an actual person, we did "the deed."

What about my Frankenboobs, you say? Have no fear; they were safely tucked away in my industrial-strength sports bra.

Word of advice: proceed with caution. Improvise. Be gentle, and, erm, flexible.

Where there's a will, there's a way...

And maybe the first time won't be the greatest sex ever. The point is the closeness, the touching, the kissing, the cuddling—it all helps you stay connected as a couple. And a couple united will probably stay that way.

A cancer diagnosis does not have to be a wedge; it can—and should—draw a couple closer together.

So a little recap: closeness; flexibility; let the small things slide; be kind to each other.

Love each other.

Exchange Surgery

All things are ready, if our mind be so.
~ *William Shakespeare, Henry V*

At my fifth saline fill, Dr. Hill decided that my previously radiated breast could take no more saline.

"The skin on the radiated side is thin," she'd say at each appointment, with a little frown.

I knew from the get-go that reconstruction via tissue expanders after radiation was speculative, but I chose the path of least resistance—i.e., shortest surgery time, shortest hospital stay, and hopefully the least amount of pain. This is not to say a woman should not undergo DIEP or TRAM flap procedures. The results from both tend to be very good. Women need to make their best informed decision after weighing the alternatives.

At this fifth appointment, Dr. Hill suggested it was time to schedule the exchange surgery. It was towards the end of October, and she proposed surgery in November, months sooner than we'd originally decided and I'd been mentally planning for. In my head, I'd gotten used to the exchange taking place sometime in the new year.

After swallowing hard a couple of times, and attempting to wrap my head around surgery right in the middle of the holiday season, I said, "Sure. Let's do it."

I'd been told and read that the permanent implants would be more comfortable than the tissue expanders since they're not so thick and tough. At this point in the process, five months out, I'd been accustomed to a tightness across my chest and pain under my right arm, radiating to the back. I wanted to feel better. Also, I was looking forward to getting rid of my freaky little Frankenboobs, which were still asymmetrical. Poor bigger-on-the-top Lefty. Poor Righty with the extra folded-under, rippled skin.

Dr. Hill flipped through her scheduling book, and we set the surgery date for November 26th, the Monday after Thanksgiving.

Yep.

I steeled myself, walked out to the waiting room to tell Steve, and looked forward to facing the new year with my surgeries behind me. I looked forward to saying goodbye to our floating year.

My Little
Patch of Miracle

**'Thank you' is the
best prayer that
anyone could say.
I say that one a lot.
'Thank you' ex-
presses extreme
gratitude, humility,
understanding.**

~ Alice Walker

When I met with the anesthesiologist for my implant exchange pre-op appointment, I made sure to mention how
sick I'd gotten from the anesthesia after my previous
three surgeries, with the last time being the worst.

"We'll give you a Scopolamine patch; that should take care of the nausea," the anesthesiologist said with confidence.

Yeah, right.

I was skeptical. I'd heard the same thing before. Would the fourth time be the charm?

On the morning of the exchange surgery, I was calmer, knowing the surgery wouldn't be as long or as traumatic to my body. While it wouldn't be a walk in the park, compared to the bilateral mastectomy and beginning reconstruction—well, actually, there *was* no comparison.

The nurse who checked me in—providing me with my hospital gown and attaching the little heater thingy so I would stay warm in the cold pre-op area—went over my health information just as before.

I decided to give it one last shot, telling her about my nausea problems and asking about the anti-nausea patch.

"Hmm, let me just check the orders," she said, squinting at her computer screen, scrolling through. "No, I don't see one ordered for you."

I sighed inwardly, hoping that my retching wouldn't be as bad as the last time. But this nurse wasn't going to let things slide. Immediately, she was on the phone taking care of business, putting in an order for the patch, and retrieving it from the dispensary a few minutes later.

She applied the patch just behind my ear, telling me I could wear it up to three days, and then I was to take it off (but to be careful not to touch my eyes after doing so because it would irritate them).

The anesthesiologist, who stopped by afterwards to check me in before surgery, also had a strategy, advising me to wait until I needed pain medication and not take the morphine but ask for a pain pill instead, which would lessen the nausea. I was a bit anxious about waiting to request pain medication—afraid of the pain, I guess—but decided to give it a go and hope for the best.

I woke up in recovery, this time not feeling much pain. Steve soon joined me after I'd already hobbled to the bathroom on my own power, accompanied by Leyna, the kind nurse who'd checked me in before my mastectomy surgery.

It was a whole different world this time. And I waited to ask for a pain pill until I needed one.

The Scopolamine patch and no morphine did the trick. For the first time in four surgeries, I didn't get sick.

Just thinking about this makes me want to turn a cartwheel, and I totally would, except I don't want my implants ending up on my back—not that they would, but this is kind of a bizarre fear of mine.

Sometimes, it's the little things.

Removing The Bandages, And Detachable Nipples

There is a thin line that separates laughter and pain, comedy and tragedy, humor and hurt.

~ Erma Bombeck

I removed my post exchange bandages after talking on the phone with Dr. Hill's nurse, prompted by her words of caution, "If you wait too long, the skin might blister."

Back in June, after my first surgery, I had a small amount of blistering when some of the bandages were left on too long. It was uncomfortable, and I wanted to avoid that happening again.

I'd missed my appointment that morning when Steve had become ill with some type of 24-hour virus. This was a problem since Dr. Hill had planned to evaluate my progress and remove most of the bandages.

At this point, a week and a half post exchange surgery, my new breasts were a maze of gauze, special foam tape which supported my new implants and helped to shape them, and steri strips over the incisions. In other words, a *lot* was going on there. And I still didn't know what my new additions looked like.

So there I stood in front of the bathroom mirror with a pail of warm water, a wash cloth, pair of scissors, and a bottle of vitamin E oil. And wine. Let us not forget that.

Slowly, I peeled back a corner of foam tape. It didn't hurt, not the *first* few millimeters. Then it did. It pulled my skin, revealing red blotches underneath. I'd grit my teeth and pull a little more, then cut the tape away, dab the skin with the wet cloth, then smooth a little oil over the area. And repeat. In some places under the foam tape, there was also clear tape. This stuff was really stuck on, and sometimes I had a hard time figuring out what was tape and what was skin. More pulling, more rubbing. This was the opposite of what we people of Earth would call a "good time."

About thirty minutes later—since I'd been proceeding slowly, wine glass handy—the bandages were gone, revealing my new breasts which were slightly asymmetrical, but not really too noticeably so. There were yellow and purple splotches here and there. The area around my underarms and the sides of my breasts was swollen with visible foam tape marks. Everything was raw looking and slightly angry.

My new breasts weren't dancing-on-the-stripper-pole large. Maybe full B cups? Perhaps a little less?

They were firmer, not like my childbirth-ravaged before-breast-cancer breasts. And they were higher up, as if I'd suddenly become many years younger. (Which is a bonus. And actually, I'm not sure if they were *ever* this high up on my body.) Each one bore a long horizontal scar* across its equator with the steri strips still in place. They would fall off eventually. (The steri strips, not my breasts.)

After my act of extreme bravery—(yes, it was very brave of me to remove my bandages myself, thank you)—my chest was a little sore and felt vulnerable since the supporting and shaping foam tape was gone.

I took a moment to pause and reflect on the past few months, knowing I could easily lapse into an emotional mess if I chose to, but I wouldn't just yet. This particular journey may have been coming to an end, but there were still areolas to tattoo. And nipples to be sewn on.

Speaking of nipples... In the days following my bilateral mastectomy and reconstruction, when my friend Sally came over for a visit, she lifted her shirt so I could see what her implants looked like now, a few years post-surgery. I'd seen her work-in-progress chest years earlier but not the finished product.

They looked good; they really did. But there were no nipples.

Where were her nipples?

She calmly explained that, yes, she *had* nipples—they'd been stitched on as part of the final cosmetic touchup procedures—but, unfortunately, one day, as she was toweling herself off after coming out of the shower, she looked down and one of them had fallen off.

One of her nipples was lying on the bathroom tile.

To repeat: *her nipple was on the floor.*

I found the idea of a detachable nipple to be: hilarious, horrifying, and slightly disturbing. But it was mostly funny, so we laughed.

I hope my eventual new nipples don't come off when I towel dry myself too enthusiastically. And I continue to await my areola tattooing process until my new breasts have healed sufficiently, the swelling has gone down enough, and Dr. Hill gives me the go-ahead.

One day, I will update my blog and share about my "finished" product.

As of this moment, I am a work in progress. But aren't we all?

*[**Tip:** *Vitamin E oil and/or Mederma Scar Cream are said to help scars fade over time. I bought a bottle of vitamin E oil at the dollar store. It lasts forever.]*

Back to Normal_ish_

Hope is the thing with feathers that perches in the soul – and sings the tunes without the words – and never stops at all.

~ *Emily Dickinson*

On March 1, 2013, I took my first court reporting job since my exchange surgery in November. My recovery had taken longer than I'd planned, mostly due to the pain in my right arm and shoulder. Since I'd been complaining to Dr. Hill at every appointment, letting her know I was still having issues, she referred me to a pain management doctor who then placed me on a low dose of Nortriptyline for what he diagnosed as muscle and possible light nerve damage. I was also referred to a physical therapist who gave me exercises and instructed me to use cold packs and a heating pad three times a day.

I needed to go back to work—for the obvious reasons most people need to work—but for also the other reasons—getting out of the house and back into the world. Getting back into some kind of a routine, some sense of normalcy and structure. I'd had enough of the amorphous floating I'd been doing. I didn't know if I was ready, though. There were fears. I'd have to lift my steno equipment and then physically perform my job duties once my equipment was all set up. It was daunting; a hurdle I'd have to clear at some point.

When I received a call at the last minute on February 28th for a short job the next morning, I swallowed a couple of times and said yes. I'd have to get back on the horse eventually.

On the drive into Los Angeles, on a much-too-warm end of winter day that felt like summer, I listened to the radio, marveled at the light Friday morning traffic, and suddenly found myself caught up in the emotion of the moment. That drive was the symbolic end of my surgery/ recovery and all it encompassed. It had been nearly one year since that day in early March of 2012 when my recurrence with breast cancer was caught. Now, I was moving forward with my life.

I fought off the tears, and sang loudly along with the radio instead.

Our Floating Year (Continues)

Go confidently in the direction of your dreams. Live the life you have imagined.

~ *Henry David Thoreau*

2012 was our floating year—Steve's, Andrew's, and mine. As I write this, in the spring of 2013, I realize that our floating year has extended. My body is still healing; I haven't returned to doing all of the things I used to be able to do, but I plan to, hopefully soon. And I still have my little cosmetic additions to "top off," if you will, my work in progress.

But it's okay.

I have been touched by the support of those I love, who've lifted me up throughout this process. The lessons I've learned from my experiences with cancer have stayed with me: life is still about the people, about the love we express for one another. We only get one shot at this; it helps to keep what matters most in perspective and not get bogged down in the trivial.

Since my first diagnosis of breast cancer, I've noticed that I cry much more easily; any display of real, honest human emotion will cause tears to well up. My emotions reside close to the surface; I'm a big, fat baby now. But that's okay, because on the flip side of the coin, I'm also quick to laugh— the sillier and more ridiculous, the better. Big, deep full-body laughs which probably exercise my abdominal muscles. A bonus!

I give thanks for the good things in life, appreciating the beauty which rises up through the common. I try to take time to see what's around me, to notice the littlest things that cross my path. I also try to distribute smiles freely and hug liberally.

These are ways cancer has transformed me.

I will strive to take the perspectives I've learned from cancer with me through the rest of my life.

I know who I am: I am a work in progress... ■

Cancer Diary: Some Things I've Learned

[I wrote this blog post on April 3, 2012, and posted it on the website Daily Kos as a diary entry. It turned into the Cancer Diaries on my blog, which turned into this book.]

If a person is going to go through something as crappy as cancer, there might as well be a lesson in there some place. (I suppose this could be the silver lining of the situation?)

When I first went through breast cancer twelve years ago, besides the initial shock, my predominating thoughts went to my beautiful two-year-old boy with his long hair and sunny disposition—just as any mother or father's would. *Would I see him grow up? How was it possible that I could be parted from him so early?* It was nearly too much to bear. I can remember the waiting—waiting on results and pathology reports; the trip to pick out the Christmas tree the same day I received my initial diagnosis, and how surreal it all was, but there was my child to be strong for, and we—Husband and I—were strong. And everything turned out just fine, which I know it will this time.

But I learned about life the first time. I became more selective about who I spent my time with. Life is too precious to spend it with energy vampires and selfish, destructive people.

I learned to give praise and compliments freely. It's not as if telling someone they look pretty today or how handsome they are in their suit will diminish your own value. Some people seem so reluctant to make others feel good about themselves, and I've never understood this.

I've also learned not to miss an opportunity to let someone know how much they mean to me or that I love them. (Okay. Maybe I'm a little mushy. Guilty.)

When someone is going through a hard time or loss, always let them know you're thinking of them. Not some clichéd platitude, but a simple "You're in my thoughts," is always appropriate. And if you say you're going to pray for someone, do. Right then. Short, sweet. But don't just say you will.

I learned twelve years ago that material goods are not so important to me. Working constantly is not where it's at. At the same time, though, I do want to travel to Paris. So there is that quandary. (Okay. I want enough money to get by, *and* I want to travel to Paris.) Paris is especially on my mind after watching *Midnight in Paris* last night. If only I could go back in time to the 1920s as main character Gil did and have one of my manuscripts critiqued by Gertrude Stein. (I wonder what she'd think about the one with the zombie teacher? I'm not sure, but she did seem like a pretty cool lady.) The writer in me loved the fantasy about nostalgia for a better time, but then Gil realizes that nostalgia is more of an escape from the present rather than the past actually being a better place. (Ain't that the truth?)

Life has been feeling very real lately. I mean, it has for a while now, but with this cancer's return, it feels even more so. I'm not as scared as I was the first time, yet I'm giving up more. My body will be forever changed.

These days, my embraces with my husband last longer; our love deepens; perspective is changed.

Our time here is short; we shouldn't waste it. (Whatever that means to you.)

Bonus Extra: The Improbability Of Christmas

[I wrote this short story five days before my bilateral mastectomy. It is not autobiographical but inspired by what I imagined a woman in my circumstance might feel.]

Everything was wrong. Nothing was right. None of it.

In the glow of the tree, Tracy reviewed her life. *It wasn't supposed to be like this.* She shook her head, despising the feel of the stubble that caused her scalp to itch all over. She felt (and probably looked) like a crazed monkey, scratching it every few seconds.

Jack had taken the Twins to a party. The thought of being separated on the holiday was, in itself, nearly impossible to grasp. But they were teens. Teens suck. There had been glimpses of humanity, though, like when Katie had set up the crèche on the side table, carefully laying out Mary, Joseph, and the baby Jesus. It had taken Tracy by surprise, this sentimental gesture, as if her usually self-absorbed sixteen-year-old daughter had been moved to keep up a family tradition. Then there was Zach, tall and lanky, with bangs that hung over his eyes. His act of kindness involved bringing the box of decorations in from the garage and placing a few things here and there around the living room as Tracy watched from her sick perch on the couch.

The two had shown periodic outward signs of compassion and team spirit. So they weren't completely evil after all.

Surgery ten days before Christmas was bad timing, but it couldn't be helped. She felt like a beached whale, still carrying twenty extra pounds from the meds, which held onto something—but what? Water weight? She hadn't eaten anything more than soup and crackers. Low-fat yogurt. Ginger ale. Air popped air.

If I'm going to pack on the poundage, shouldn't I be eating coconut cream pies topped with hot fudge?

She shook her head again, catching a glimpse of the macaroni and glitter ornament with Katie's wide eyes and smile beaming back at her. Zach's counterpart hung on the branch underneath. The sight of their childhood goodness made her catch her breath.

The trip to pick out the tree had been a major effort.

"Come on, Mom," Zach urged. "You can do it."

"It's too soon," she said in protest, trying to beg off. It had only been eight days post-surgery, and the pain meds weren't as fun as she'd hoped. And they'd had the disappointing effect of making her feel loopy *and* constipated. It still felt as if a pile of bricks were sitting squarely on top of her empty chest.

Jack put his hand on her shoulder, delicately, always with care, and said softly, "Come on, Babe. You can sit in the car."

Little steps. Each one pushing her ever-so-slightly forward.

She sat on the couch; her family gone. Everything had changed. Time had passed. The excited laughter that had once sounded like tinkly silver bells had been replaced by deep guffaws and ironic jokes. She looked at the scene of the Holy Family and pondered the improbability of the Christ child—a delicate baby born in a smelly, crowded manger still remembered over two thousand years later. She considered the improbability of her husband still finding her attractive with her ashy complexion and extra weight. Hell, she had no hair *and* was missing parts. Two, to be specific. And they were key parts. Lovemaking would never be quite the same again. She still couldn't look at herself.

She sighed and watched as the family's golden Labradoodle strolled over to the middle of the living room floor and began to make that familiar heaving motion.

"Oh, no. Don't do it," she pleaded.

He did do it. All over the wood floor.

"Dammit, Judd Nelson!"

He'd been named as an inside joke, but his viscous ooze was anything but. Tracy heaved herself off of the couch, dragged into the kitchen, ripped a few paper towels from the roll and, slowly, carefully, lowered herself down to the floor to clean.

"What a mess. I'm a mess," she said to her dog. He showed an appalling lack of concern and sat scratching himself.

As she slowly wiped, she thought of Jack, back twenty years when they'd met as art majors. He was shy, had the bluest of blue eyes, smiled easily, and told terrible jokes. He'd show up in drawing class and give her strange and wonderful gifts, like the time he'd carved a shriveled-up apple man, or the Easter Island head he whittled from a king-sized bar of Ivory soap. She'd kept it to this day. It sat on her dresser, and she'd give it a little pat now and then when she'd pass by.

There were picnics in the park where they'd lie on the grass and talk about their plans for the future–the hopes and dreams that any young couple would have— about how one day they'd get a little apartment by the beach and sell their paintings on the pier.

But money, or lack thereof, had a way of making life hard and mean. Work for artists was difficult to come by in the new Digital Age with jobs being shipped overseas and everyone and their monkey doing their own desktop "art." Jack worked in a home supply store. Retail hell.

It wasn't supposed to be like this.

She dragged herself up off of the hardwood floor and gave Judd Nelson a pat on the head.

"Don't do that again, please."

He ran off to check his food dish, and she held the wet paper towels, dropping them in the kitchen trash, catching sight of herself in the mirror. She brought a hand up, touching her face. The gauntness in combination with her hair stubble caught her off guard.

How can he love me like this?

That was perhaps the most improbable of all thoughts. Jack was still handsome. His hair was a little thinner, and he'd gained a few pounds around the middle, but he was healthy and strong. *It's not fair for him. He's left with this?* She looked down at her extra fat roll and thought of her husband with a younger, more attractive wife. *Bastard!* Then she laughed at herself, having broken her own rule, which was: You can't get mad at people when they disappoint you in hypothetical situations, or dreams.

She made her way back onto the couch and called for her dog.

"Come here, Judd, you big dummy. Keep me company. It's Christmas Eve."

Even though he was eighty pounds of lazy, he jumped onto the couch in a flash, and Tracy let his infraction slide, the couch normally being off limits to dog sorts. He shoved his nose in her face, and she stroked his fur, feeling a tad less crappy about life but in no less pain. They sat for a few moments until Judd's ears perked, his attention drawn to the front door. He hopped off to greet his master who had returned from ferrying the kids to their party.

"Hello, beautiful," Jack said, touching her shoulder and leaning down for a kiss.

The touch was warm; the kiss lingered on her lips. She kissed him back, and there was nothing about it that suggested it was perfunctory or obligatory. The kiss encompassed years together; years to come.

Jack pulled his face away from hers. She saw his smile, his blue eyes with the crinkly skin at the edges, and knew that one day they'd be chasing each other around the retirement home's Christmas tree, using their walkers.

Everything was as it should be.

Acknowledgements:

I thank my doctors, nurses, and technicians responsible for my care these past thirteen years, and thank you to Kaiser Permanente Southern California for not skimping with my treatment. Thank you to my editor Ellen Brock for excellent and thorough work, and to my husband and partner-in-life Steve for the cover design as well as interior layout of this book, also for his valuable input and suggestions. (There are not enough thank yous for Steve.) Thank you to Laura Goodman and Marian Carter for your input, suggestions, and general feedback. Thank you to Andrew for being a great kid throughout it all. And thank you to my mother, my mother-in-law, my sisters, my brother Jon who we miss terribly, and my friends, online and off, for having my back and holding me up. I love you all.

My Backers:

[This book was made possible by the generosity of my Kickstarter backers. You all gave this project its wings, and because of your financial and moral support, you gave me the strength to do this. I simply cannot thank you all enough.]

- **Christopher Blydenburgh** in honor of his mother, Elaine Blydenburgh

- **Jonas Ritter**

- **Monica Tackes Dawson**

- **Beth Bowland** in honor of the "Fabulous Webster Women"

- **Joe Herman**

- **Jeff Winbush**

- **Crystal Dolan**

- **Nancy Gordon** in memory and in honor of Melinda Gordon

- **Elizabeth Jouvenat** in honor of family and friends affected by cancer
- **Jennifer Carter** in memory of Jon
- **Melinda** in memory of her dad, Dean L. Taylor
- **Carolyn Sandoval**
- **Mary Chmura**
- **Anonymous donor**
- **PK** in honor of Marg
- **Rhea Rhodan**
- **Catia Cecilia Confortini** in honor of her mother, Martina Moladori
- **Big Al Crowntown**
- **Kathy Miller** for Margaret in honor of her journey
- **Bonnie Lundin**
- **Bridget Gieseke** in gratitude for being healthy for the last six years!
- **Pamela** *and* **Kerby Mellott** in gratitude for Ethan
- **Karen Burton** in memory of George Pompey
- **Laura Goodman** in honor of known friends and unknown friends who have suffered from breast cancer
- **Rose Lucero** in honor of Tricia Cobb and Margaret Carter, the two bravest women I know
- **Sharon Ledwith** in memory of Carmen Molnar
- **Jennifer Murphy**

Very Special Thank You To My Squirrels; The Super Backers:

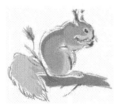

- **Michele Owens** in memory of her grandmother, Ida Skelly

- **Mary**

- **Elaine** *and* **Bobby Cowley** in honor of Cris Kelly

- **Theresa** in honor of old friends and new

- **Sue Lesh**

- **Karen** in honor of Margaret Lesh and in recognition of her phenomenal positive attitude!

- **Marian Carter**

- **The Fisher Girls—Tammie, Kimmie, Billie Jo,** *and* **Jennifer**

- **Eric** *and* **Violet Mandeson**

- **Kevin Van Lierde** in honor of his mom

- **Carol Lynne Brown-Wilson** in memory of Grandpa Rex Brown, Grandma Helen Brown-Mantooth, Rex Alan Brown, Michelle Meere, Uncle Jim Carter, Cousin Jon Carter, Phil and Loreen Brown, Cousin Phillip Brown, Grandma and Grandpa DuPass, Aunt Sharon Cooper, Nancy Irving Rhodes, Brian James, Elephant Mike Sullivan, and Steve Fuller, *and* in honor of Renee Stevens

About The Author:

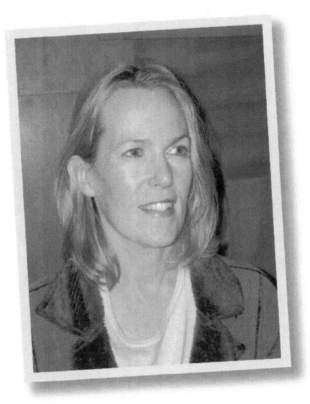

Margaret Lesh is a freelance court reporter and author of the novels *Normalish* and *Finding a Man for Sylvia*. She lives in Southern California with her art director husband and teen son. They make her laugh almost every day. She has a special relationship with tacos and baked goods.

Buy her books on Amazon.com (or Barnes & Noble or iBooks or at your local thrift store):

Normalish:

- http://www.amazon.com/dp/B009LTC8Z6
  Fifteen-year-old Stacy questions the strange world of high school, family, friends, love, and her role in the universe.

Finding A Man For Sylvia:

- http://www.amazon.com/dp/B00ABUTN2K
  A well-intentioned but clueless romantic is determined to find love for her lonely neighbor over her exasperated husband's objections.

Visit her website:

- http://margaretlesh.com

Read her blog (you'll like this):

- http://storyrhyme.com/jcsblog

She tweets too:

- https://twitter.com/margaretlesh

Made in the USA
San Bernardino, CA
21 July 2015